Keto Low Carb Diet For Beginners

*Healthy and Delicious Ketogenic Diet Recipes
to Lose Weight and Feel Great
with the Low Carb Diet*

Anne Spencer

CONTENTS

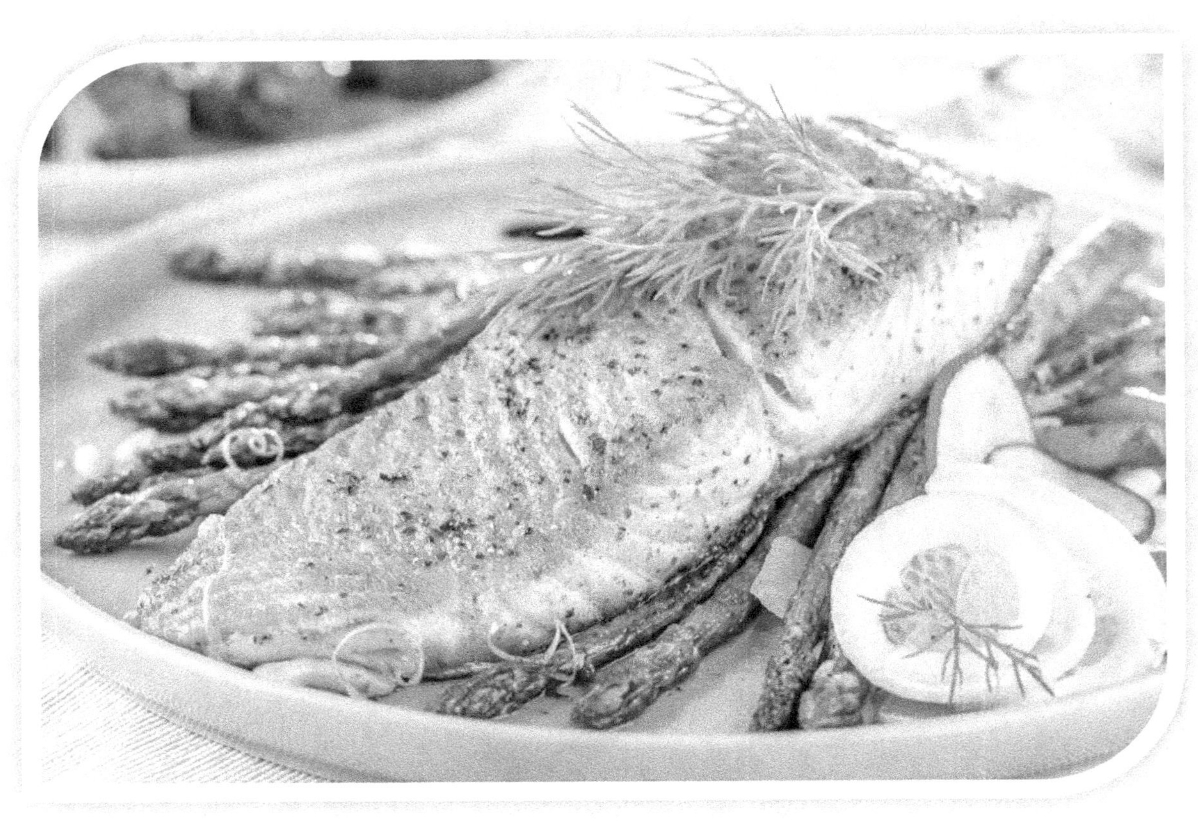

INTRODUCTION

It's widely-spread knowledge that our bodies are designed to run primarily on carbs. We use them to provide our bodies with the energy required to boost our state, exercise, or just normal body functioning. However, most people are clueless about the fact that carbs are not the only source of fuel our bodies can use. Just like they can run on carbs, our bodies can also use fat sources. When we ditch the carbs and focus on providing our bodies with more fat, we are embarking on the ketogenic train.

The ketogenic diet is not just another fad diet. It has been around since 1920 and has resulted in outstanding results and amazingly successful stories. If you are new to the keto world and have no idea what I am talking about, let me simplify this for you.

For you to truly understand what the keto diet is all about and why you should start it as soon as you can, let me first explain what happens to your body after consuming a carb-loaded meal.

Imagine you have just swallowed a giant bowl of spaghetti. Your tummy is full, your taste buds are satisfied, and your body is provided with more carbs than necessary. After consumption, your body immediately starts the process of digestion, during which your body will break down the consumed carbs into glucose, which is a source of energy your body depends on. So one might ask, "What is wrong with carbs?" For starters, there are some things: they raise the blood sugar, make your body work excessively to offset the effects of that sugar, and kindly storing it as another layer of fat, usually around the belly, but many times around the organs too. That's extremely dangerous. Sounds scary? I know.

By now, you've undoubtedly heard of the keto diet and the many people who have had success losing weight and keeping it off. But just what is a ketogenic diet, and how does it work to reach your weight loss goal.

The keto diet is a food plan that is high in fat and low in carbs. The human body uses carbohydrates as its primary fuel source; however, when fats replace carbs, the body enters a metabolic state known as "ketosis." During

ketosis, because of the lack of carbs, the body will burn stored fat as fuel, which can help you lose weight.

Not only can the keto diet promote weight loss, but it also comes with numerous health benefits:

- Management of diabetes
- Lower cholesterol
- Improved mental clarity
- Reduces the risk and symptoms of polycystic ovary syndrome (POS)
- Lower risk of some cancers
- Lower risk of cardiovascular disease

The keto diet requires a change in your wearing habits. It's easier to make these changes when you have your partner or other family members' active support. As a couple, you'll be able to encourage each other on those days that are more difficult than others for sticking to your food plan.

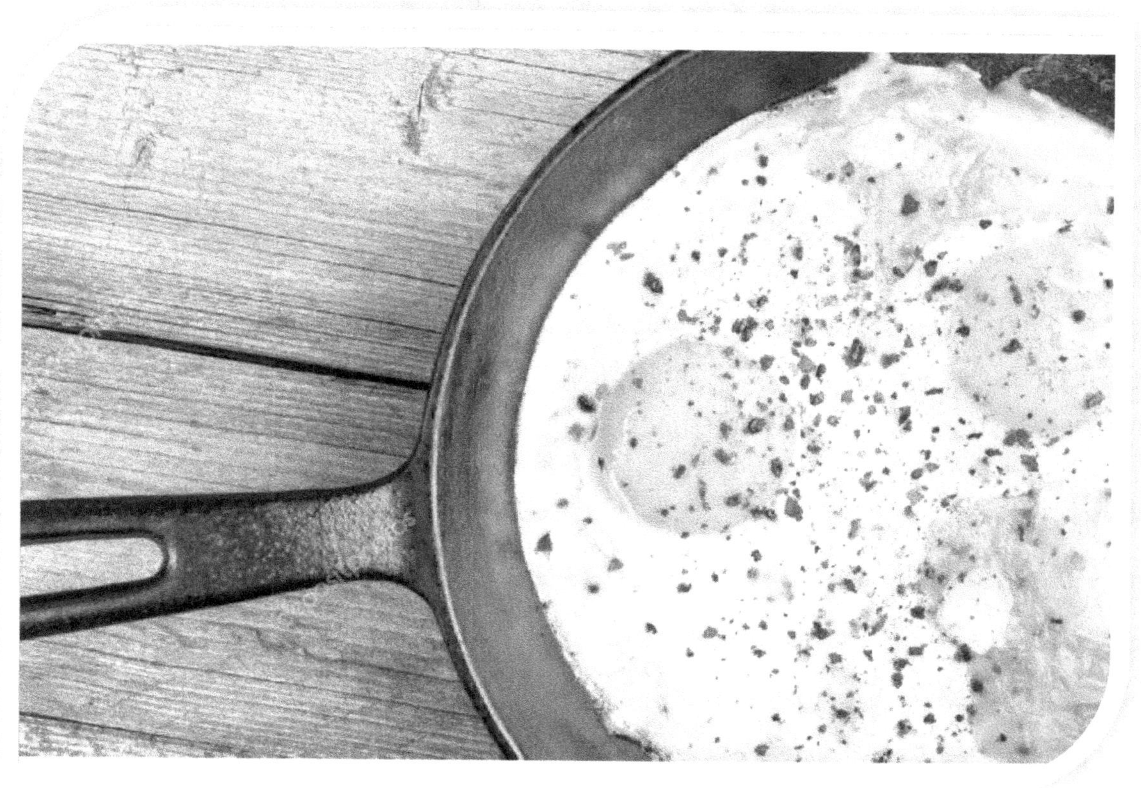

THE KETOSIS

Switching to high fat moderate protein cycle, your liver now has a new "fuel boss" - the fat. Once your liver begins preparing your body for the fuel change, the fat from the liver will start producing ketones – hence the name Ketogenic. What glucose is for the carbs, the ketones are for the fat, meaning they are the tiny molecules created once the fat is broken down to be used as energy. The switch from glucose to ketones is something that has pushed many people away from this diet. Some people consider this to be a dangerous process, but the truth is, your body will run just as efficiently on ketones as it does on glucose.

Once your body shifts to using ketones as fuel, you are in the state of ketosis. Ketosis is a metabolic process that may be interpreted as a little 'shock' to your body. However, this is far from dangerous. Every change in life requires adaptation, and so does this. This adaptation process is not set in stone, and every person goes through ketosis differently. However, for most people, it takes around 2 weeks to adapt to the new lifestyle fully.

Note! This is all biological and completely healthy. You have spent your whole life packing your body with glucose; naturally, you need time to adapt to the new dietary change.

Foods Allowed On the Keto Diet

Plan your meals and snacks around the following foods:

- Eggs
- Meats, including beef, pork, chicken, and veal
- Fish, including fish high in fat such as mackerel, trout, and salmon
- Cheeses
- Nuts and seeds, including nut and seed butter

* Cream and butter

* Avocadoes

* Healthy oils, such as olive, avocado, and coconut oils

* Low-carb vegetables, such as peppers, onions, tomatoes, and green vegetables

* Herbs and spices, including salt and pepper

To be sure you're getting enough of the right nutrients, eat a wide variety of meats, vegetables, seeds, and nuts on the allowed food list.

Foods Restricted On the Keto Diet

These are the foods that are restricted on a ketogenic food plan:

* Grains and starches, such as bread, pasta, cereal, and rice

* Carrots, potatoes, yams, sweet potatoes, and parsnips

* Beans and legumes, including chickpeas, lentils, and peas

* Fruit, except for small quantities of berries

* Sugar in any form, including foods that contain fructose

* Processed diet foods and Alcohol

* Condiments that contain sugar

* Unhealthy fats, such as processed vegetable oils and mayonnaise

* Alcohol

Getting Started with Your Keto Diet

Before starting the keto diet, take some time researching the foods on the allowed list and those restricted foods. Plan your meals ahead of time and shop accordingly, filling your kitchen with keto-friendly foods.

Healthy snacks

To make it easier to stick to the keto diet, it's important to have healthy snacks. If you're on the keto diet with your partner, have keto-approved snacks on hand that you both enjoy. Approved snacks include:

- Hard-boiled eggs, cheese, and olives
- A handful of nuts and seeds
- Celery and red pepper sticks with guacamole and salsa
- No-sugar plain yogurt mixed with berries

Intermittent Fasting and the Keto Diet

Intermittent fasting is all about restricting the number of calories you consume within a period so that you put your body into a "fasted" state. When this happens, the body's insulin levels will start to lower, which increases the fat burning process.

The Benefits of Intermittent Fasting Include:

- Weight loss
- Improved mental clarity
- Management and reducing the risk of type 2 diabetes
- Lower risk of cardiovascular disease
- Lower risk of some cancers

The most common fasting method is to fast each day for 14 to 16 hours, restricting the time you eat to a "window" of 8 to 10 hours. During the eating window, you should be eating at least 2 to 3 healthy keto meals. An excellent way to approach intermittent fasting is eating your last meal by 8 pm on any day and not eating your first meal until midnight the next day.

Another intermittent fasting method includes the 5:2 rule, where you only eat 500 to 600 calories per day on two days of the week, eating a healthy keto diet for the other five days. Another fasting method is the eat-stop-eat plan, where you fast for 24 hours twice a week.

Both intermittent fasting and the keto diet put the body into a ketosis state to use up stored fat for energy. When you combine intermittent fasting with the keto diet, you may be able to put your body into ketosis faster than dieting alone. This can lead to faster and more efficient weight loss.

What to Expect on the Keto Diet & Keto "Flu"

During the first few days of starting the Keto, you may experience an increase in hunger, lack of energy, and problems sleeping. Some people may also experience nausea and digestive issues. These flu-like symptoms are known as the "keto flu." To alleviate these symptoms, consider doing a low-carb diet for a week slowly transitioning into the full keto diet. During the first month, always eat until you feel full without focusing on restricting calories. Ease into the food plan, so you're less likely to stop eating a ketogenic diet.

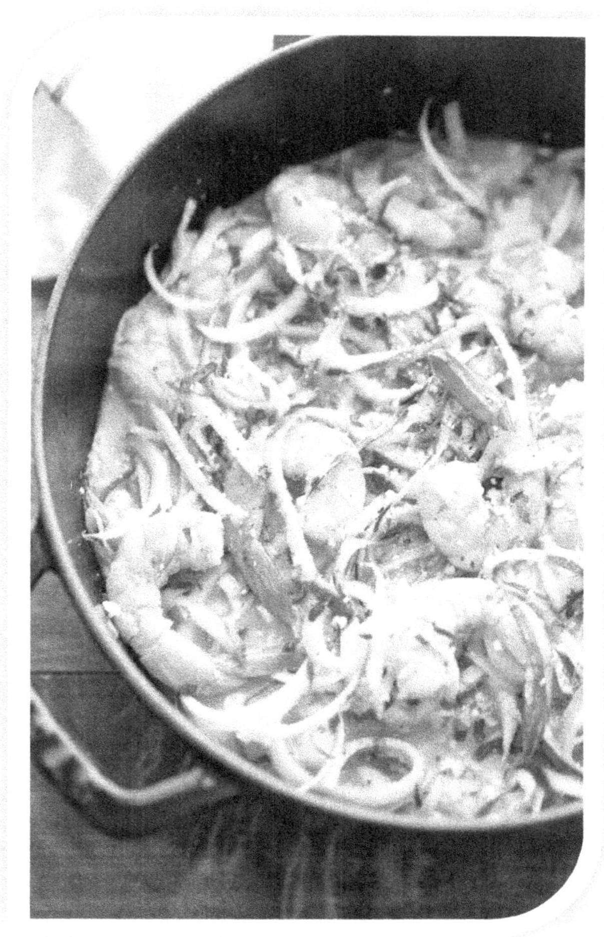

The keto diet changes the mineral and water balance of your body. Make sure that you're drinking more water each day. As well, taking a mineral supplement and adding a bit of extra salt to your diet can keep help maintain a healthy balance of minerals and water, helping to relieve any of the flu-like symptoms. For a mineral supplement, take 300 mg of magnesium and 1,000 mg of potassium.

DIET – THE NEW LIFESTYLE

The Benefits of Keto Diet

Even though it is still considered 'controversial,' the keto diet is the best dietary choice one can make. From weight loss to longevity, here are the benefits that following a ketogenic diet can bring to your life:

Loss of Appetite

You can't tame your cravings? Don't worry. While on ketosis, you won't feel exhausted or with a rumbling gut. The keto diet will help you say no to that second piece of cake. Once you train your body to run on fat and not on carbs, you will experience a drop in appetite that will work magic for your figure.

Weight Loss

Since the body is forced to produce only a small amount of glucose, it will lower insulin production. When that happens, your kidneys will start getting rid of the extra sodium, which will lead to weight loss.

HDL Cholesterol Increase and Drop in Blood Pressure

While consuming a diet high in fat and staying clear of harmful glucose, your body will experience a rise in good HDL cholesterol levels, which will, in turn, reduce the risk for many cardiovascular problems. Cutting back on carbs will also drop your blood pressure. The drop in blood pressure can prevent many health problems such as strokes or heart diseases.

Lower Risk of Diabetes

Although this probably goes without saying, it is essential to mention this one. When you ditch the carbs, your body is forced to lower the glucose productivity significantly, which leads to a lower risk of diabetes, including a reverse in the condition if you already have it.

Improved Brain Function

Many studies have shown that replacing carbohydrates with fat as an energy source leads to mental clarity and improved brain function. This is yet another reason why you should go Keto.

Should You Try the Keto Diet?

The keto diet can help you lose weight and keep it off. When you're eating nutritiously, exercising, and following a ketogenic food plan, you'll be joining the many other people around the world who have successfully lost weight.

Whether you're starting the keto diet on your own or as a couple, begin with the keto food plan basics to become familiar with the foods you can and can't eat. As you start to lose weight and learn how to customize your meals, the keto diet plan will become a natural part of your lifestyle, allowing you to maintain your health and weight loss.

BASIC & SIMPLE RECIPES

1. AVOCADO A LA CARBONARA

Ingredients

For 4 servings

- 2 eggs, beaten
- 1 ½ cups cream cheese
- 5 ½ tbsp psyllium husk
- 1 avocado, peeled and pitted
- 1 ¾ cups coconut cream
- Juice of ½ lemon
- 1 teaspoon onion powder
- ½ teaspoon garlic powder
- ¼ cup olive oil
- Salt and black pepper to taste
- ¼ cup grated Parmesan
- 4 tbsp toasted pecans

Directions

Total Time: approx. 30 minutes

1. Preheat oven to 300 F. In a bowl, add the eggs, cream cheese, psyllium husk, and salt to taste. Whisk until smooth batter forms. Line a baking sheet with wax paper, pour in the batter, and cover with another wax paper. Use a rolling pin to flatten the dough into the sheet. Bake for 12 minutes, then take off the wax papers and slice the "pasta" into thin strips lengthwise.

2. Cut each piece into halves, pour into a bowl, and set aside. In a blender, combine avocado, coconut cream, lemon juice, onion and garlic powders and puree until smooth. Pour olive oil over the "pasta" and stir to coat. Pour the avocado sauce on top and mix well. Sprinkle with salt, pepper, and freshly grated Parmesan cheese. Garnish with toasted pecans and serve.

Per serving:

- Cal 769
- Net Carbs 8g
- Fat 56g
- Protein 35g

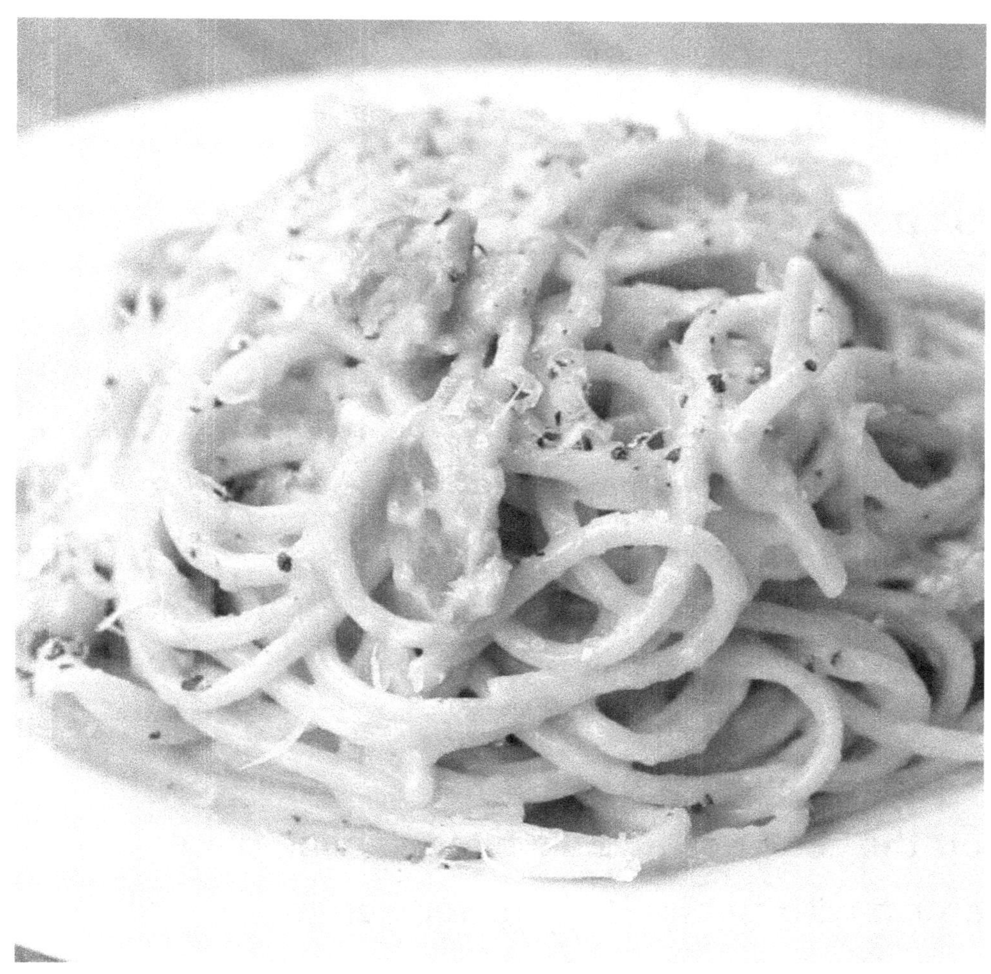

2. GOLDEN SAFFRON CAULI RICE

Ingredients

For 4 servings

- A pinch of saffron soaked in ¼-cup almond milk
- 1 tbsp butter
- 2 tbsp olive oil
- 6 garlic cloves, sliced
- 1 yellow onion, thinly sliced
- 2 cups cauli rice
- ¼ cup vegetable broth
- 2 tbsp chopped parsley
- Salt and black pepper to taste

Directions

Total Time: approx. 15 minutes

1. Warm olive oil in a saucepan over medium heat and fry garlic until golden brown but not burned; set aside.
2. Sauté butter and onion in the saucepan for 3 minutes. Stir in cauli rice.
3. Remove the saffron from the milk and pour the milk and stock into the saucepan.
4. Mix, cover, and cook for 5 minutes. Season with salt, black pepper, and parsley.
5. Fluff the cauli rice and dish into serving plates.
6. Garnish with the fried garlic and serve.

Per serving:

- Cal 89
- Net Carbs 5.9g
- Fat 6g
- Protein 2g

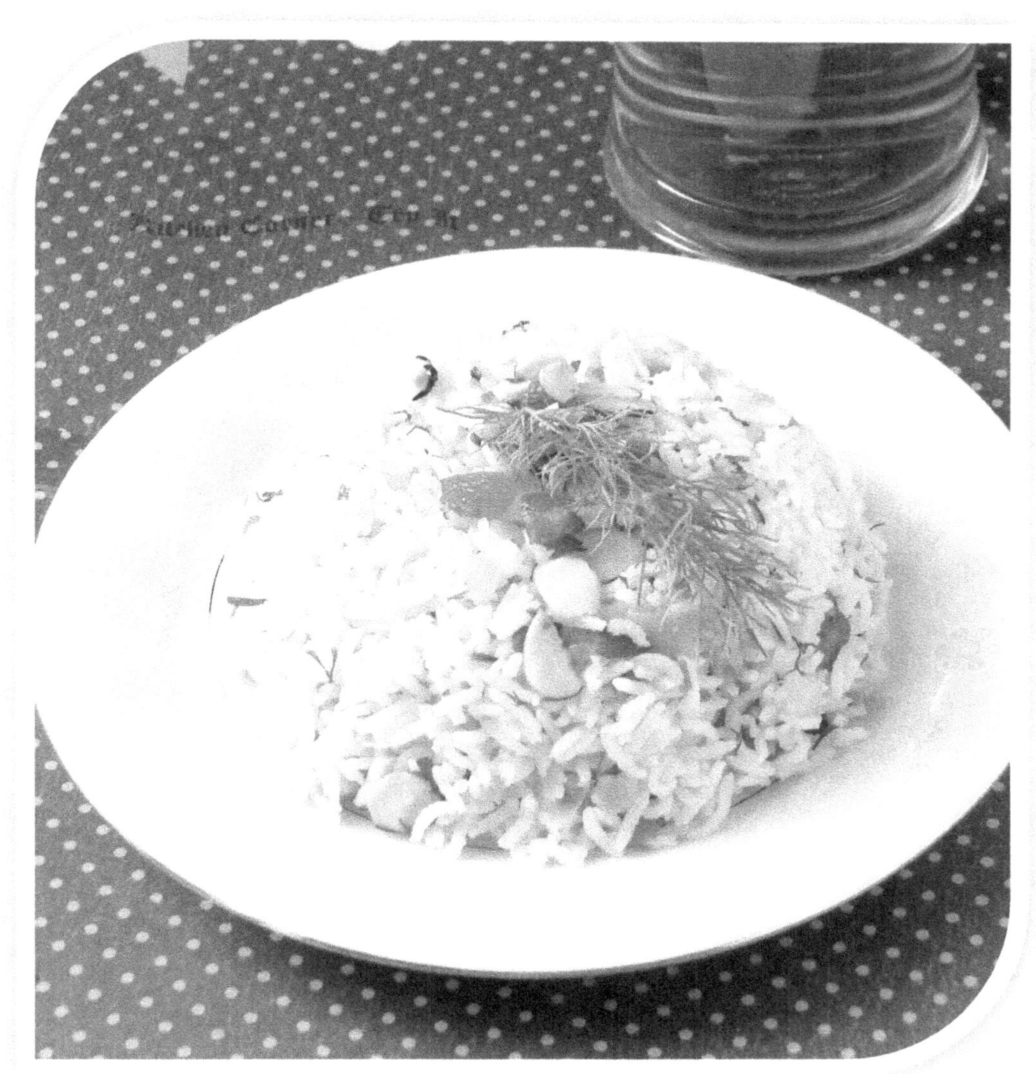

BREAK FAST & EGGS

3. ALMOND & RASPBERRIES CAKES

Ingredients

For 4 servings

- 2 cups almond flour
- 2 tsp baking soda
- 1 tsp vanilla extract
- 2 tbsp almond flakes
- ½ tsp salt
- 2 tbsp liquid stevia
- 8 oz cream cheese, softened
- ¼ cup butter, melted
- 1 egg
- 10 raspberries
- 1 cup almond milk

Directions

Total Time: approx. 35 minutes

1. Mash the raspberries with a fork and set aside.
2. Mix the almond flour, baking soda, vanilla, and salt in a large bowl. In a separate bowl, whisk the egg and almond milk.
3. Add in the cream cheese, stevia, and butter and beat until well incorporated.
4. Fold in the flour and mashed raspberries and spoon the batter into greased muffin cups two-thirds way up.
5. Top with almond flakes.

6. Bake for 20 minutes at 400 F until golden brown, remove to a wire rack to cool slightly for 5 minutes before serving.

Per serving:

- Cal 353
- Fat 33g
- Net Carbs 8.6g
- Protein 9.4g

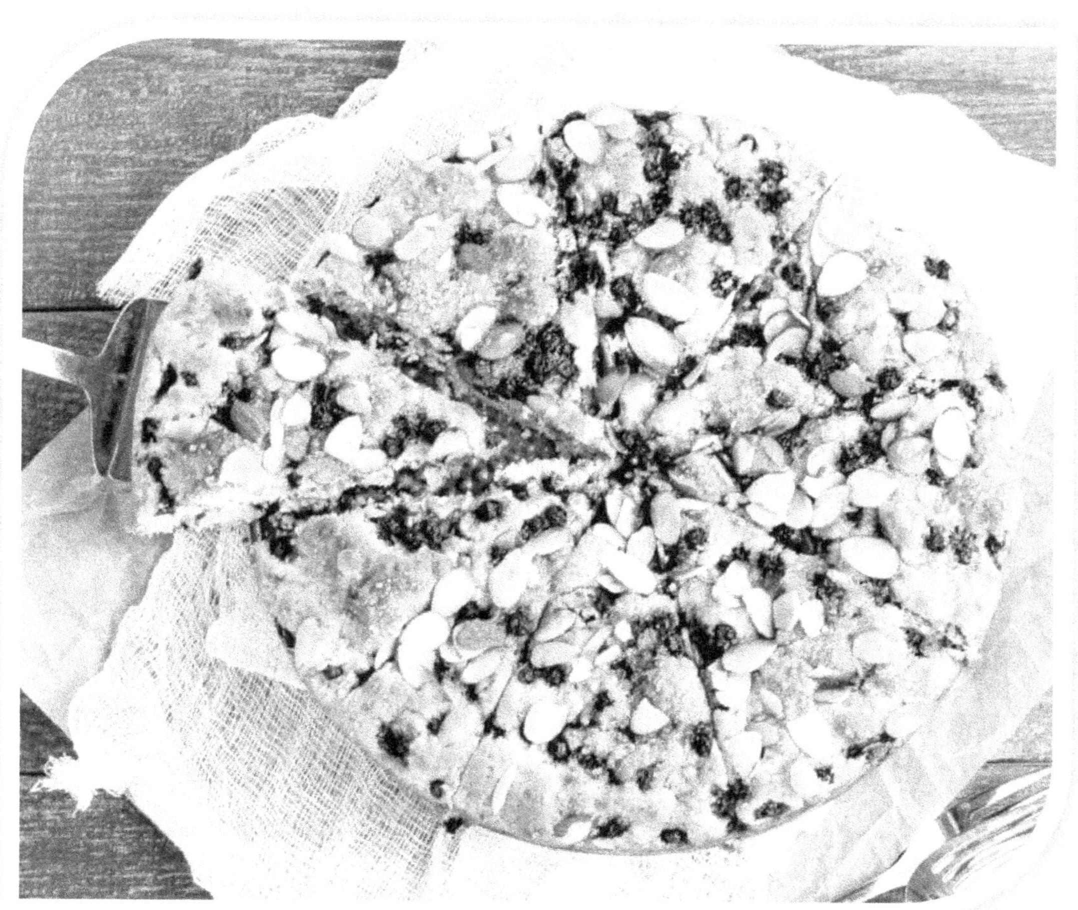

4. BACON & BLUE CHEESE CUPS

Ingredients

For 4 servings

- 2 tbsp olive oil
- 6 eggs
- 2 tbsp coconut milk
- Salt and black pepper to taste
- ½ cup blue cheese, crumbled
- 4 oz bacon, chopped
- 2 tbsp chives, chopped
- 1 serrano pepper, minced

Directions

Total Time: approx. 30 minutes

Preheat oven to 390 F. Beat the eggs in a bowl and whisk in coconut milk until combined. Season with salt and pepper; fold in the blue cheese.

Grease muffin cups with olive oil and spread the bottom of each one with bacon. Fill each with the egg mixture two-thirds way up. Top with serrano pepper and bake in the oven for 18 minutes or until golden. Remove and allow cooling for a few minutes. Serve topped with chives.

Per serving:

- Cal 354
- Fat 28g

- Net Carbs 1.5g

- Protein 24g

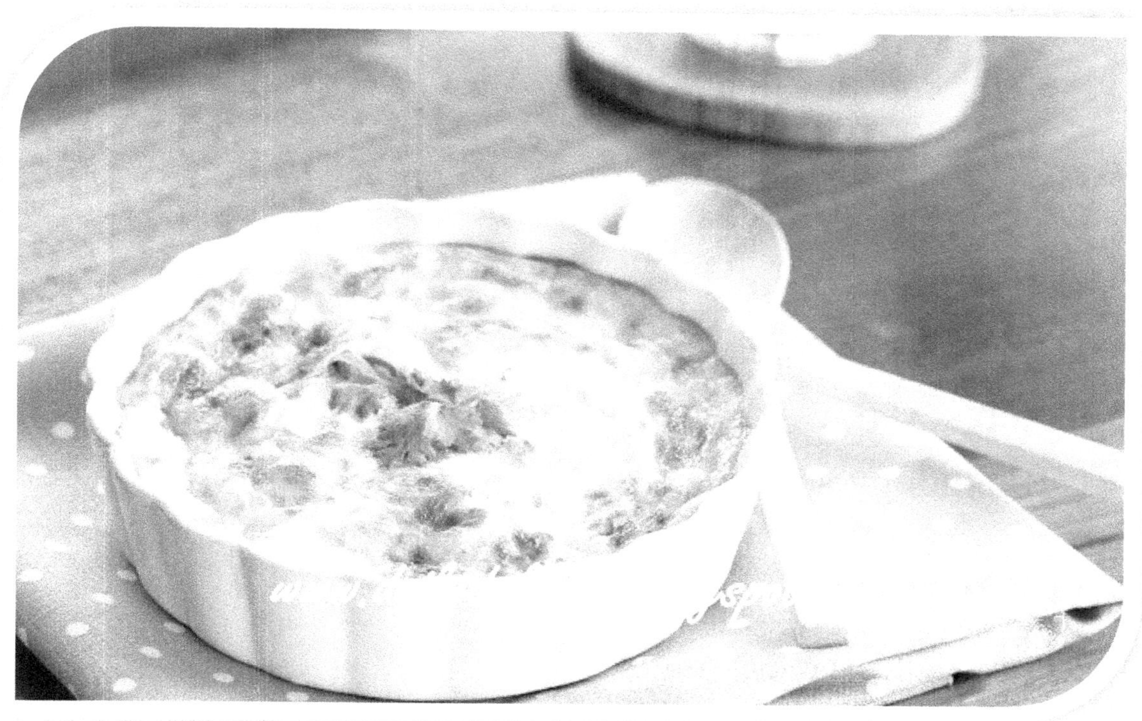

5. SESAME & POPPY SEED BAGELS

Ingredients

For 4 servings

- ½ cup coconut flour
- 6 eggs
- ½ cup flaxseed meal
- ½ tsp onion powder ½ tsp garlic powder
- 1 tsp dried oregano
- 1 tsp sesame seeds
- 1 tsp poppy seeds

Directions

Total Time: approx. 30 minutes

1. Mix the coconut flour, eggs, ½ cup of water, flaxseed meal, onion powder, garlic powder, and oregano.
2. Spoon the mixture into a greased donut tray. Sprinkle with poppy seeds and sesame seeds.
3. Bake the bagels for 20 minutes at 360 F.
4. Let cool for 5 minutes before serving.

Per serving:

- Cal 431
- Fat 20g
- Net Carbs 1.3g
- Protein 29g

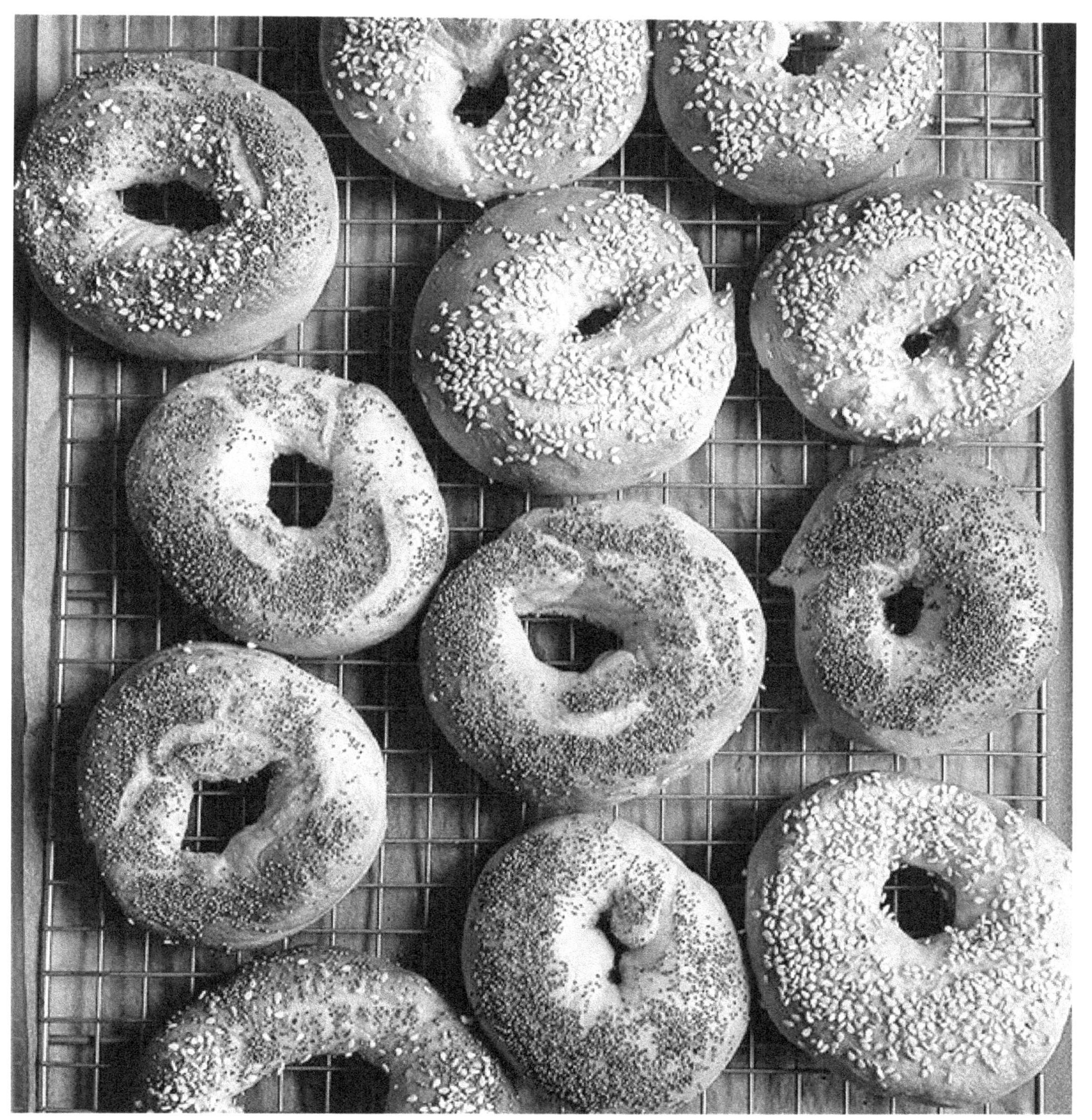

SALADS & SOUPS

6. ARUGULA & WATERCRESS TURKEY SALAD

Ingredients

For 4 servings

- 1 tbsp xylitol
- 1 red onion, chopped
- 2 tbsp lime juice
- 3 tbsp olive oil
- 1 ¾ cups raspberries
- 1 tbsp Dijon mustard
- Salt and black pepper, to taste
- 1 cup arugula
- 1 cup watercress
- ½ lb turkey breasts, boneless
- 4 oz goat cheese, crumbled
- ½ cup walnut halves

Directions

Total Time: approx. 25 minutes

1. Start with the dressing: In a blender, combine xylitol, lime juice, 1 cup raspberries, pepper, mustard, ¼ cup water, onion, olive oil, and salt and pulse until smooth.
2. Strain this into a bowl and set aside.
3. Heat a pan over medium heat and grease lightly with cooking spray.

4. Coat the turkey with salt and black pepper and cut in half.

5. Place skin side down into the pan.

6. Cook for 8 minutes, flipping to the other side and cooking for 5 minutes.

7. Place arugula and watercress in a salad platter, scatter with the remaining raspberries, walnut halves, and goat cheese.

8. Slice the turkey, put over the salad, and top with raspberries dressing to serve.

Per serving:

- Cal 511
- Fat 35g
- Net Carbs 7.5g
- Protein 37g

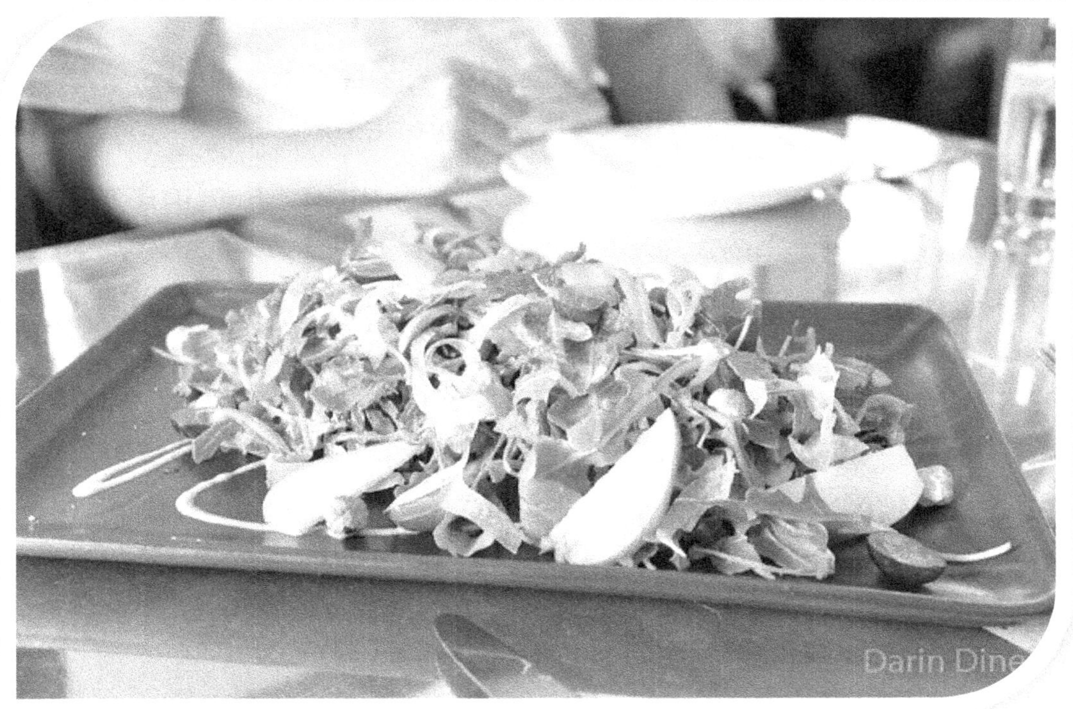

7. SPINACH SALAD WITH GOAT CHEESE & NUTS

Ingredients

For 2 servings

- 2 cups spinach
- ½ cup pine nuts
- 1 cup hard goat cheese, grated
- 2 tbsp white wine vinegar
- 2 tbsp extra virgin olive oil
- Salt and black pepper, to taste

Directions

Total Time: approx. 20 min + cooling time

1. Preheat oven to 390 F. Place the grated goat cheese in two circles on two parchment paper pieces.
2. Place in the oven and bake for 10 minutes. Find two same bowls, place them upside down, and carefully put the parchment paper on top to give the cheese a bowl-like shape. Let cool that way for 15 minutes. Divide spinach among the bowls, sprinkle with salt and pepper, and drizzle with vinegar and olive oil. Top with pine nuts to serve.

Per serving:

- Cal 410
- Fat 32g
- Net Carbs 3.4g

- Protein 27g

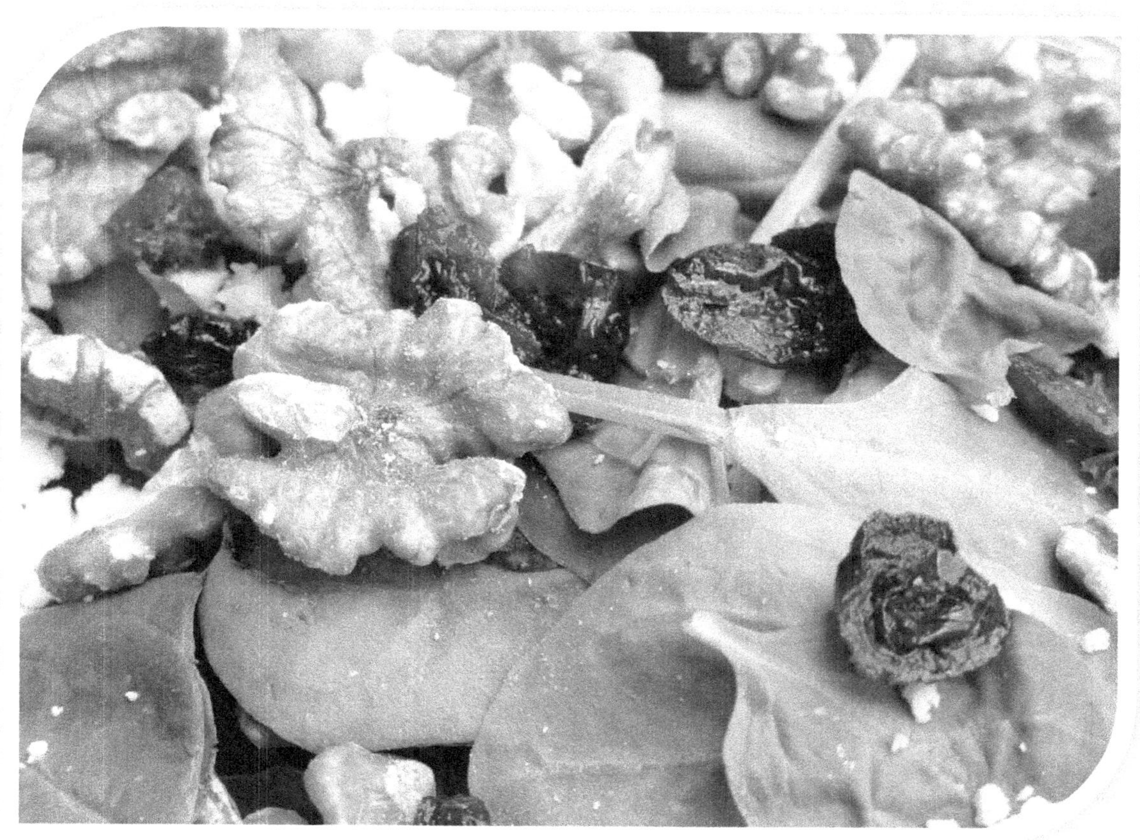

8. THAI-STYLE PRAWN SALAD

Ingredients

For 2 servings

- 2 cups watercress
- 1 green onion, sliced ½ lb prawns, cooked
- 1 avocado, sliced
- 1 Thai chili pepper, sliced
- 1 tomato, sliced
- 1 tbsp cilantro, chopped
- ¼ tsp sesame seeds
- 1 tbsp lemon juice
- 2 tsp liquid stevia
- ½ tsp fish sauce
- 1 tbsp sesame oil

Directions

Total Time: approx. 20 minutes

1. In a bowl, whisk the stevia, sesame oil, fish sauce, and lemon juice.
2. Add the prawns and toss to coat.
3. Refrigerate covered for 10 minutes. Combine watercress, avocado, tomato, Thai chili pepper, and green onion on a serving platter.
4. Top with prawns and drizzle the marinade over.
5. Sprinkle with sesame seeds and cilantro and serve.

Per serving:

- Cal 420
- Fat 29g
- Net Carbs 1.8g
- Protein 29g

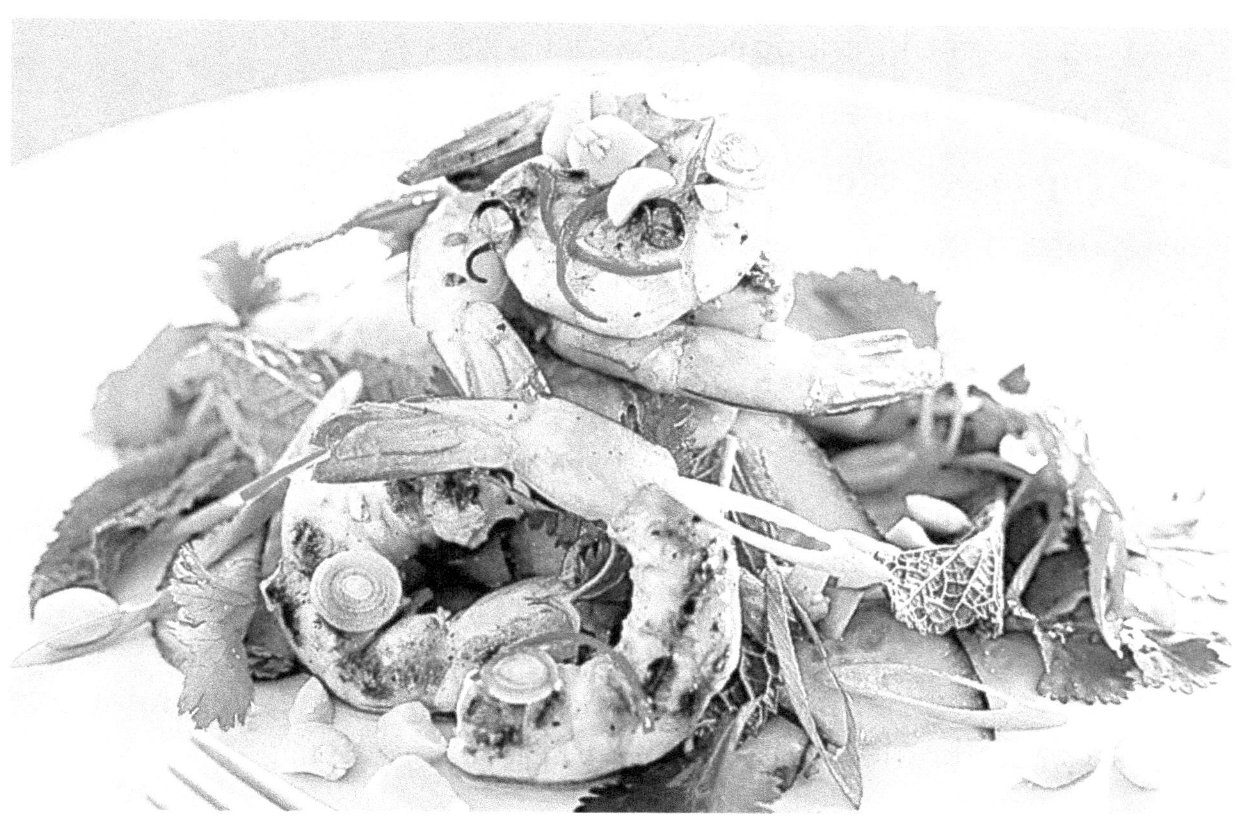

9. CREAM OF CAULIFLOWER & LEEK SOUP

Ingredients

For 4 servings

- 4 cups vegetable broth
- 16 oz cauliflower florets
- 1 celery stalk, chopped
- 1 onion, chopped
- 1 cup leeks, chopped
- 2 tbsp butter
- 1 tbsp olive oil
- 1 cup heavy cream
- ½ tsp red pepper flakes

Directions

Total Time: approx. 45 minutes

1. Warm butter and olive oil in a pot set over medium heat and sauté onion, leeks, and celery for 5 minutes.
2. Stir in the broth and cauliflower and bring to a boil; simmer for 30 minutes.
3. Transfer the mixture to an immersion blender and puree; add in the heavy cream and stir.
4. Decorate with red pepper flakes and serve.

Per serving:

- Cal 255
- Fat 21g
- Net Carbs 5.3g
- Protein 4.4g

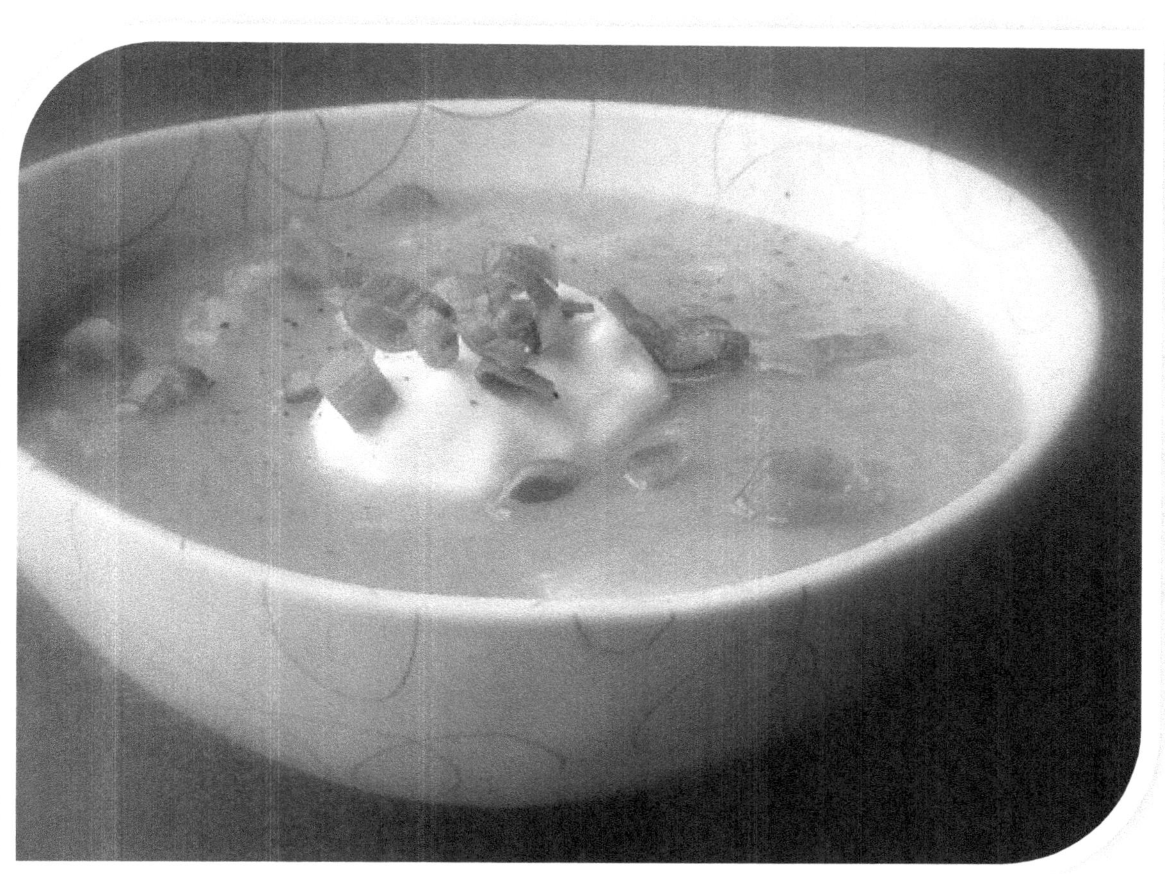

POULTRY

10. CHICKEN "FOUR CHEESES "WITH PANCETTA

Ingredients

For 4 servings

- 1 lb chicken breasts
- 4 oz mozzarella cheese, cubed
- ¼ cup mascarpone cheese
- ¼ cup cheddar cheese, cubed
- 4 oz provolone cheese, cubed
- 1 green bell pepper, sliced
- Salt and black pepper, to taste
- 1 oz pancetta, sliced

Directions

Total Time: approx. 45 minutes

1. Fry pancetta in a pan over medium heat until crispy, 5 minutes. Set aside to cool, then crush it.

2. In a bowl, mix together bell pepper and crushed pancetta. Stir in mascarpone, cheddar cheese, provolone cheese, and mozzarella cheese.

3. Cut slits into chicken breasts, season with black pepper and salt and stuff with the cheese mixture.

4. Set on a lined baking sheet Bake in the oven at 400 F for 30 minutes.

Per serving:

- Cal 355
- Fat 23g
- Net Carbs 2.2g
- Protein 33g

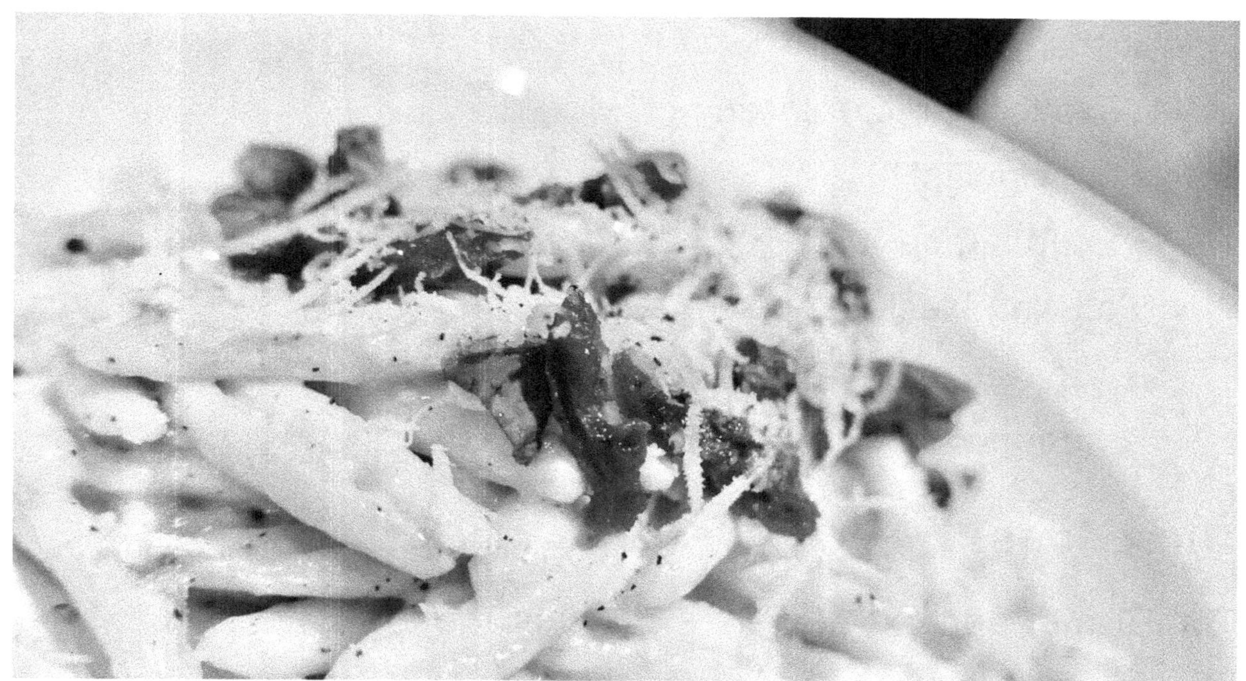

11. CHICKEN SOUVLAKI

Ingredients

For 2 servings

- 1 red bell pepper, cut into chunks
- 2 chicken breasts, cubed
- 2 tbsp olive oil
- 2 cloves garlic, minced
- 8 oz cipollini
- ½ cup lemon juice
- Salt and black pepper to taste
- 1 tsp rosemary, chopped
- 2 lemon wedges to garnish

Directions

Total Time: approx. 20 min + chilling time

1. In a bowl, mix half of the oil, garlic, salt, pepper, and lemon juice and add the chicken, cipollini, and bell pepper.
2. Marinate for 2 hours in the fridge.
3. Preheat a grill to high heat.
4. Thread chicken, bell pepper, and cipollini onto skewers and grill them for 6 minutes on each side.
5. Remove and serve garnished with rosemary and lemons wedges.

Per serving:

- Cal 363

- Fat 14g

- Net Carbs 4g

- Protein 32g

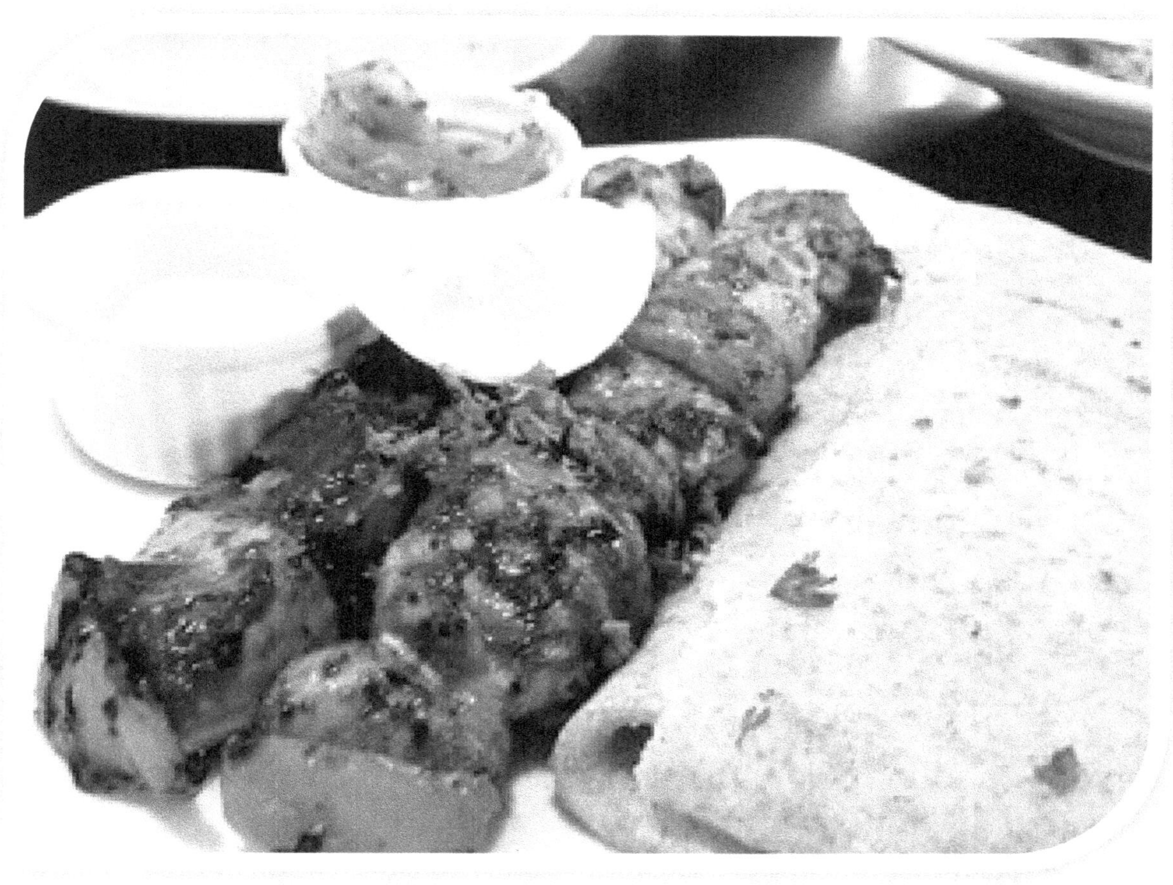

12. TEXAS CHICKEN SLIDERS

Ingredients

For 4 servings

- 1 lb chicken thighs, boneless and skinless
- 2 zero carb hamburger buns, halved
- ½ cup chicken broth
- ¼ cup melted butter
- ¼ cup baby spinach
- 4 slices cheddar cheese
- 1 tsp onion powder
- 2 tsp garlic powder
- 1 tbsp ranch dressing mix
- ¼ cup white vinegar
- 2 tbsp hot sauce
- Salt and black pepper to taste

Directions

Total Time: approx. 1 hour 15 minutes

1. Place a pot over low heat and add vinegar, hot sauce, broth, and butter.
2. In a bowl, combine onion and garlic powders, salt, pepper, and ranch dressing mix.
3. Rub the mixture onto the chicken and place it into the pot.
4. Cook for 1 hour. Shred the chicken into small strands with two forks. Adjust the taste.

5. Divide the spinach on the bottom half of each zero-carb bun, spoon the chicken on top, and add a cheddar cheese slice.

6. Cover with the remaining bun halves and serve.

Per serving:

- Cal 781
- Net Carbs 15g
- Fat 41g
- Protein 92g

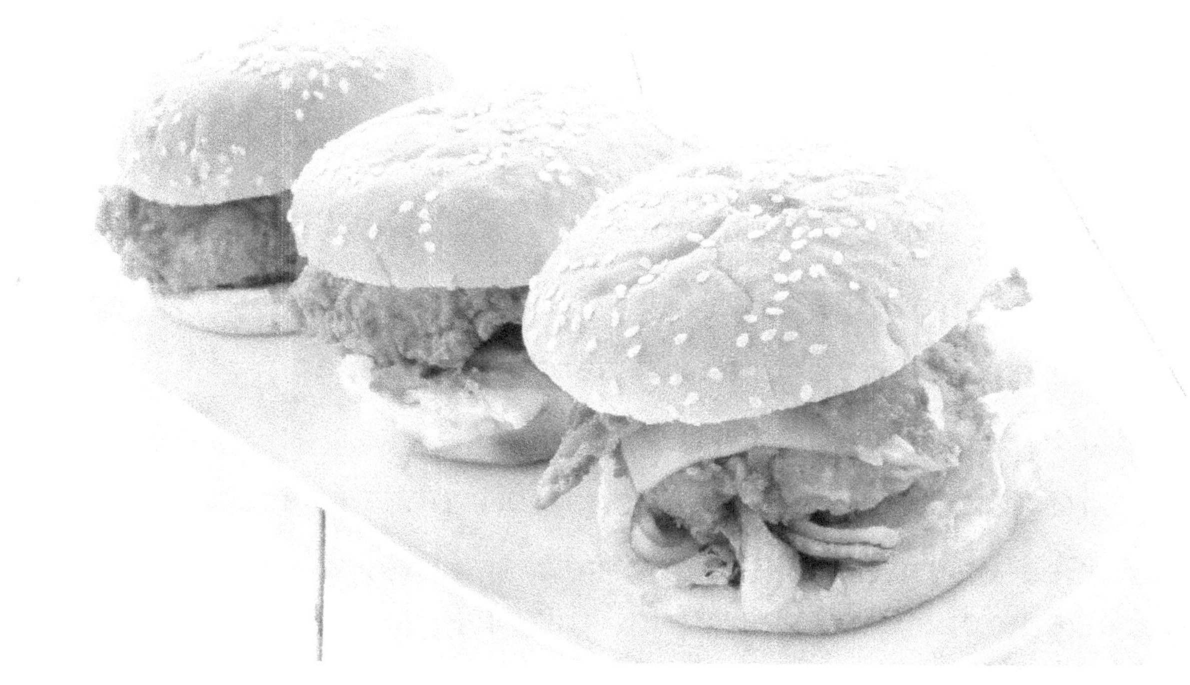

13. BAKED CHEESY CHICKEN TENDERS

Ingredients

For 4 servings

- 1 tbsp olive oil
- 2 eggs
- 3 cups crushed cheddar cheese
- ½ cup pork rinds, crushed
- 1 lb chicken tenders
- Salt to taste
- Lemon wedges for garnish

Directions

Total Time: approx. 45 minutes

1. Preheat oven to 370 F.
2. Line a baking sheet with parchment paper.
3. Beat the eggs in a bowl.
4. Mix the cheddar cheese and pork rinds in another bowl.
5. Season the chicken with salt, dip in egg mixture, and coat generously in cheese/rind mixture.
6. Place on the baking sheet, cover with aluminium foil and bake for 25 minutes.
7. Remove foil, brush with olive oil, and bake further for 10 minutes until golden brown.
8. Serve chicken with lemon wedges.

Per serving:

- Cal 512
- Fat 43g
- Net Carbs 2.2g
- Protein 35g

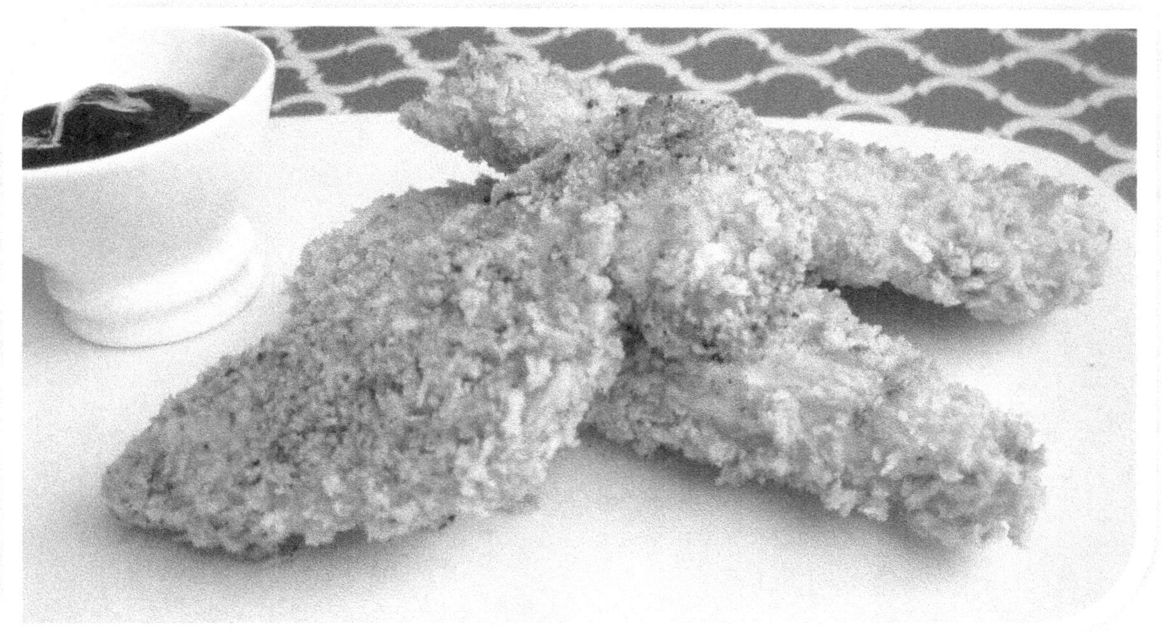

BEEF & LAMB

14. BELL PEPPERS STUFFED WITH ENCHILADA BEEF

Ingredients

For 6 servings

- 3 tbsp butter, softened
- 6 bell peppers, deseeded
- ½ white onion, chopped
- 3 cloves garlic, minced
- 2 ½ lb ground beef
- 3 tsp enchilada seasoning
- 1 cup cauliflower rice
- ¼ cup grated cheddar cheese
- Sour cream for serving
- Salt and black pepper to taste

Directions

Total Time: approx. 60 minutes

1. Preheat oven to 380 F.
2. Melt butter in a skillet over medium heat and sauté onion and garlic for 3 minutes.
3. Stir in beef, enchilada seasoning, salt, and pepper.
4. Cook for 10 minutes.
5. Mix in the cauli rice until well incorporated.

6. Spoon the mixture into the peppers, top with the cheddar cheese, and put the stuffed peppers in a greased baking dish.

7. Bake for 40 minutes.

8. Drop generous dollops of sour cream on the peppers and serve.

Per serving:

- Cal 411
- Net Carbs 4g
- Fat 19g
- Protein 48g

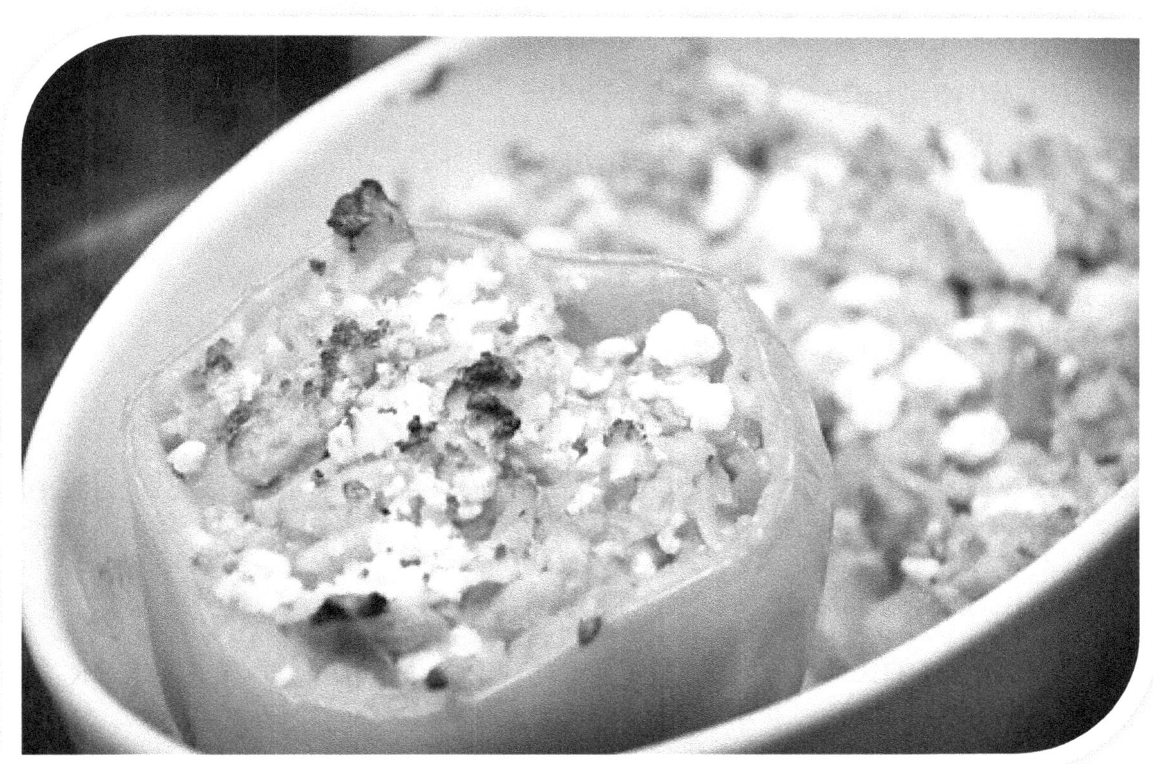

15. LETTUCE CUPS WITH SPICY BEEF

Ingredients

For 4 servings

- 3 tbsp ghee, divided
- 1 lb chuck steak
- 1 large white onion, chopped
- 2 garlic cloves, minced
- 1 jalapeño pepper, chopped
- 2 tsp red curry powder
- 1 cup cauliflower rice
- 8 small lettuce leaves
- Salt and black pepper to taste
- ¼ cup sour cream for topping

Directions

Total Time: approx. 30 minutes

1. Warm 2 tbsp of the ghee in a large deep skillet.
2. Sliced the beef thinly against the grain and cook until brown and cooked within, 10 minutes; set aside.
3. Sauté the onion in the skillet for 3 minutes.
4. Pour in garlic, salt, pepper, and jalapeño and cook for 1 minute.
5. Add the remaining ghee, curry powder, and beef.
6. Cook for 5 minutes and stir in the cauliflower rice.

7. Sauté until adequately mixed and the cauliflower is slightly softened, 2 to 3 minutes.

8. Adjust the taste with salt and pepper.

9. Lay out the lettuce leaves on a lean flat surface and spoon the beef mixture onto the middle part of them, 3 tbsp per leaf.

10. Top with sour cream, wrap the leaves, and serve.

Per serving:

- Cal 302

- Net Carbs 3.3g

- Fat 21g

- Protein 32g

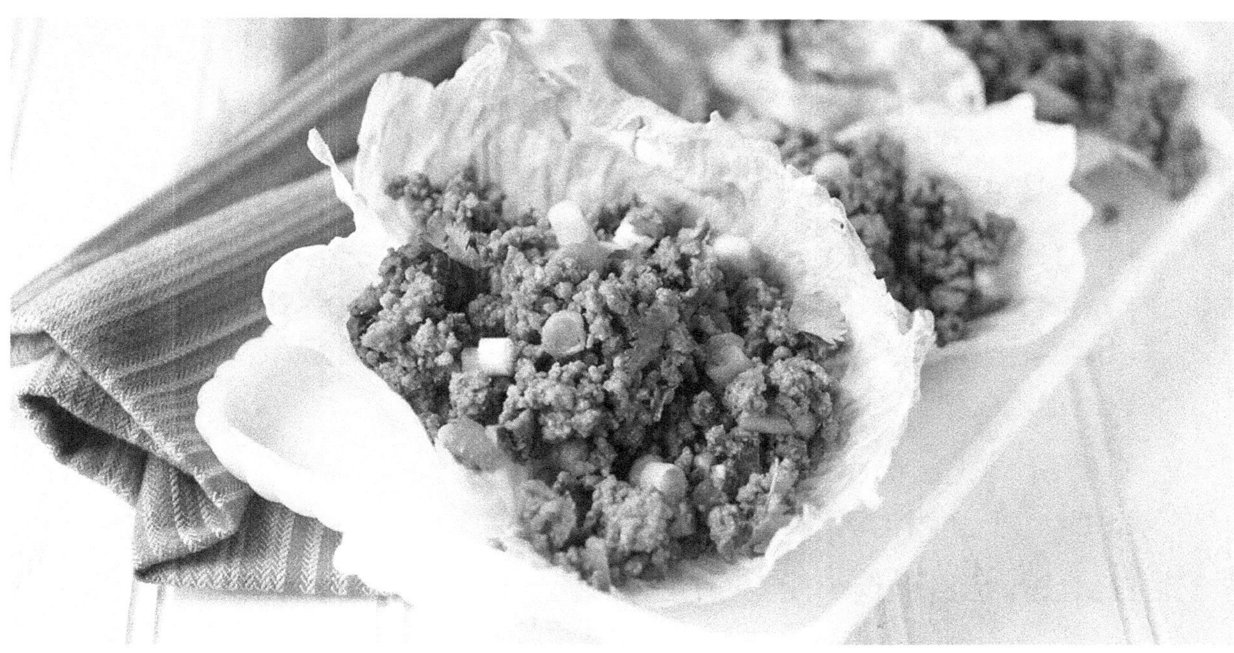

16. BASIL BEEF SAUSAGE PIZZA

Ingredients

For 4 servings

- 2 tbsp butter
- 2 tbsp cream cheese, softened
- 10 oz shredded mozzarella
- 8 oz ground beef sausage
- 1 egg
- ¾ cup almond flour
- 1 tsp plain vinegar
- ¼ cup tomato sauce
- ½ tsp dried basil

Directions

Total Time: approx. 50 minutes

1. Preheat oven to 390 F. Line a pizza pan with parchment paper. Melt the cream cheese and half of the mozzarella cheese in a skillet over low heat while stirring until evenly combined.

2. Turn the heat off and mix in almond flour, egg, and vinegar. Let cool slightly.

3. Flatten the mixture onto the pizza pan.

4. Cover with another parchment paper and, using a rolling pin, smoothen the dough into a circle.

5. Take off the parchment paper on top, prick the dough all over with a fork and bake for 10 to 15 minutes until golden brown.

6. While the crust bakes, melt butter in a skillet over and fry sausage until brown, 8 minutes.

7. Turn the heat off. Spread the tomato sauce on the crust, top with basil, meat, and remaining mozzarella cheese, and return to the oven.

8. Bake for 12 minutes. Remove the pizza, slice, and serve.

Per serving:

- Cal 359
- Net Carbs 0.8g
- Fat 19g
- Protein 41g

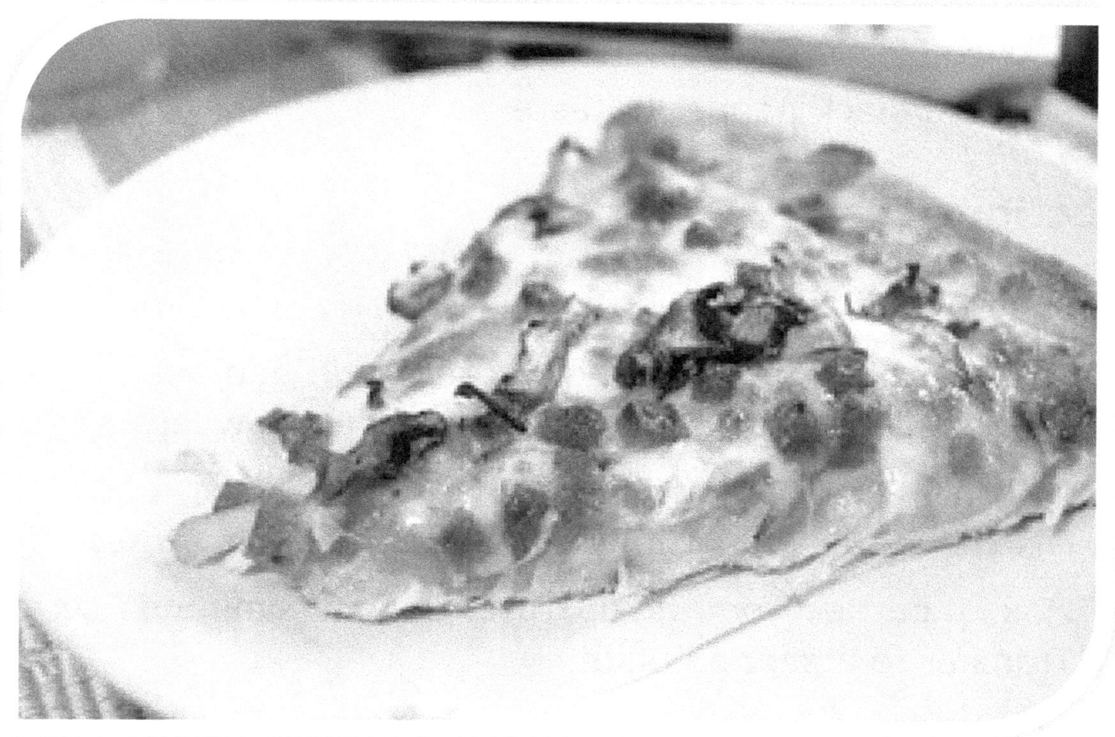

17. SPINACH CHEESEBURGERS

Ingredients

For 4 servings

- 1 lb ground beef
- 4 tomato wedges, deseeded
- ½ cup chopped cilantro
- 1 lemon, zested and juiced
- 1 tsp garlic powder
- 2 tbsp hot chili puree
- 16 large spinach leaves
- 4 tbsp mayonnaise
- 1 medium red onion, sliced
- ¼ cup grated Parmesan
- 1 avocado, halved, sliced
- Salt and black pepper to taste

Directions

Total Time: approx. 15 minutes

1. Preheat the grill to high heat. In a bowl, add beef, cilantro, lemon zest, juice, salt, pepper, garlic powder, and chili puree.
2. Mix the ingredients until evenly combined.
3. Make 4 patties from the mixture. Grill for 3 minutes per side. Transfer to a serving plate.
4. Lay 2 spinach leaves side to side in 4 portions on a clean flat surface.

5. Place a beef patty on each and spread 1 tbsp of mayo on top.

6. Add a slice of tomato and onion, sprinkle with some Parmesan, and place avocado on top.

7. Cover with 2 pieces of spinach leaves each.

8. Serve the burgers with cream cheese sauce.

Per serving:

- Cal 308
- Net Carbs 6.5g
- Fat 16g
- Protein 31g

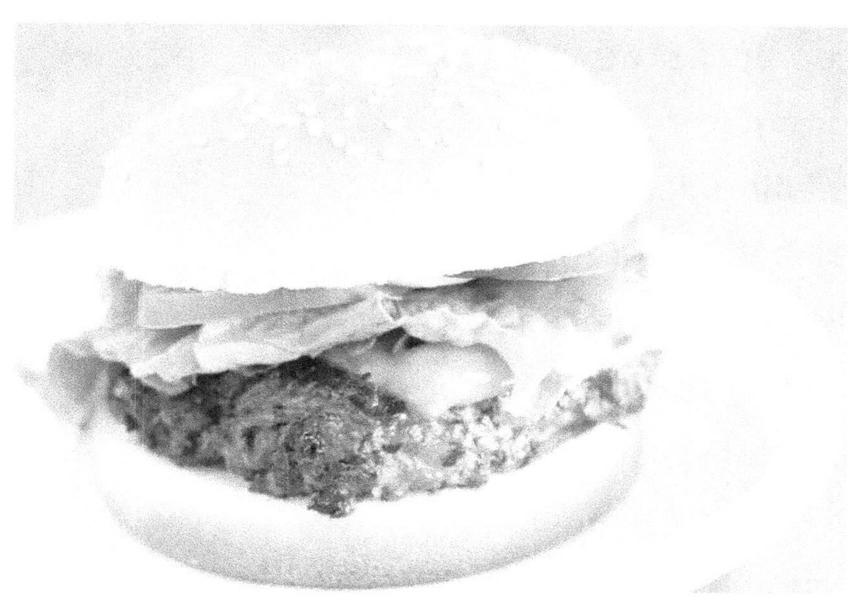

18. BEEF PAD THAI WITH PEANUTS & ZUCCHINI

Ingredients

For 4 servings

- 3 large eggs, lightly beaten
- 2 ½ lb chuck steak
- 1 tsp red pepper flakes
- 1 tsp pureed garlic
- ¼ tsp freshly ground ginger
- 1 tbsp peanut oil
- 2 ¼ tbsp peanut butter
- 1 /3 cup beef broth
- 2 tbsp tamari sauce
- 1 tbsp white vinegar
- ½ cup chopped green onions
- 1 garlic cloves, minced
- 4 zucchinis, spiralized
- ½ cup bean sprouts
- ½ cup crushed peanuts
- Salt and black pepper to taste

Directions

Total Time: approx. 30 minutes

1. Using a sharp knife, slice the beef thinly against the grain. In a bowl, combine garlic puree, ginger, salt, and pepper. Add in beef and toss to coat.

2. Heat peanut oil in a deep skillet and cook the beef for 12 minutes; transfer to a plate. Pour the eggs into the skillet and scramble for 1 minute; set aside. Reduce the heat and combine broth, peanut butter, tamari sauce, vinegar, green onions, minced garlic, and red pepper flakes.

3. Mix until adequately combined and simmer for 3 minutes. Stir in beef, zucchini, bean sprouts, and eggs. Cook for 1 minute. Garnish with peanuts.

Per serving:

- Cal 433

- Net Carbs 3.3g

- Fat 38g

- Protein 69g

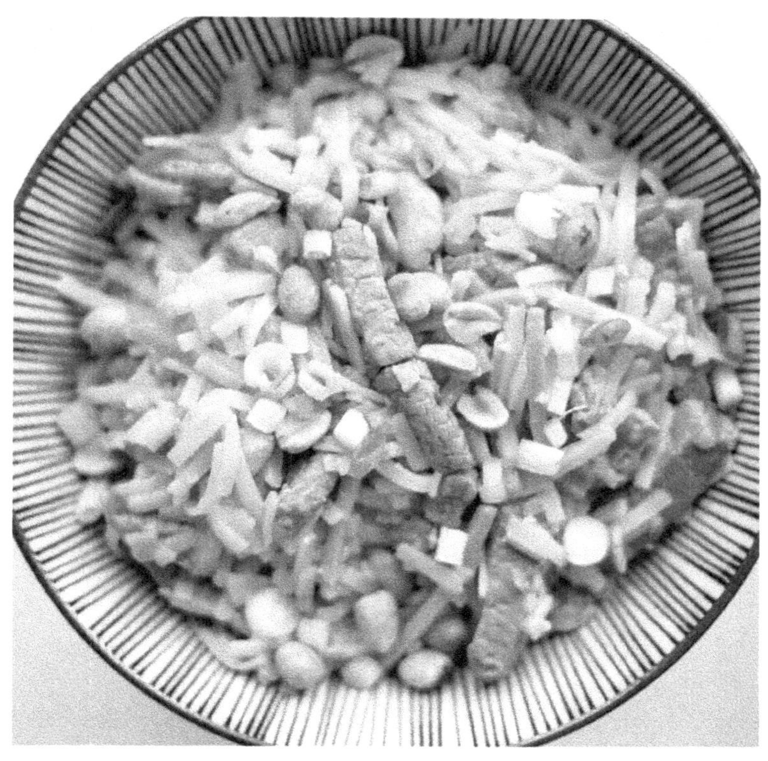

FISH & SEAFOOD

19. QUICK TUNA OMELET

Ingredients

For 2 servings

- 1 avocado, sliced
- 1 tbsp chopped chives
- 1 /3 cup canned tuna, drained
- ¼ tsp smoked cayenne pepper
- 4 eggs, beaten
- 4 tbsp mascarpone cheese
- 1 tbsp butter
- Salt and black pepper, to taste

Directions

1. Total Time: approx. 15 minutes
2. Melt the butter in a pan over medium heat.
3. Pour in the eggs and cook for 3 minutes.
4. Flip the omelet and continue to cook for 2 more minutes or until golden.
5. Sprinkle with cayenne pepper, salt and pepper.
6. Slide the omelet onto a plate and spread the mascarpone cheese over.
7. Top with tuna, avocado, and chives.
8. Fold the omelet in half to cover the filling and serve.

Per serving:

- Cal 481
- Fat 38g
- Net Carbs 6.2g
- Protein 279g

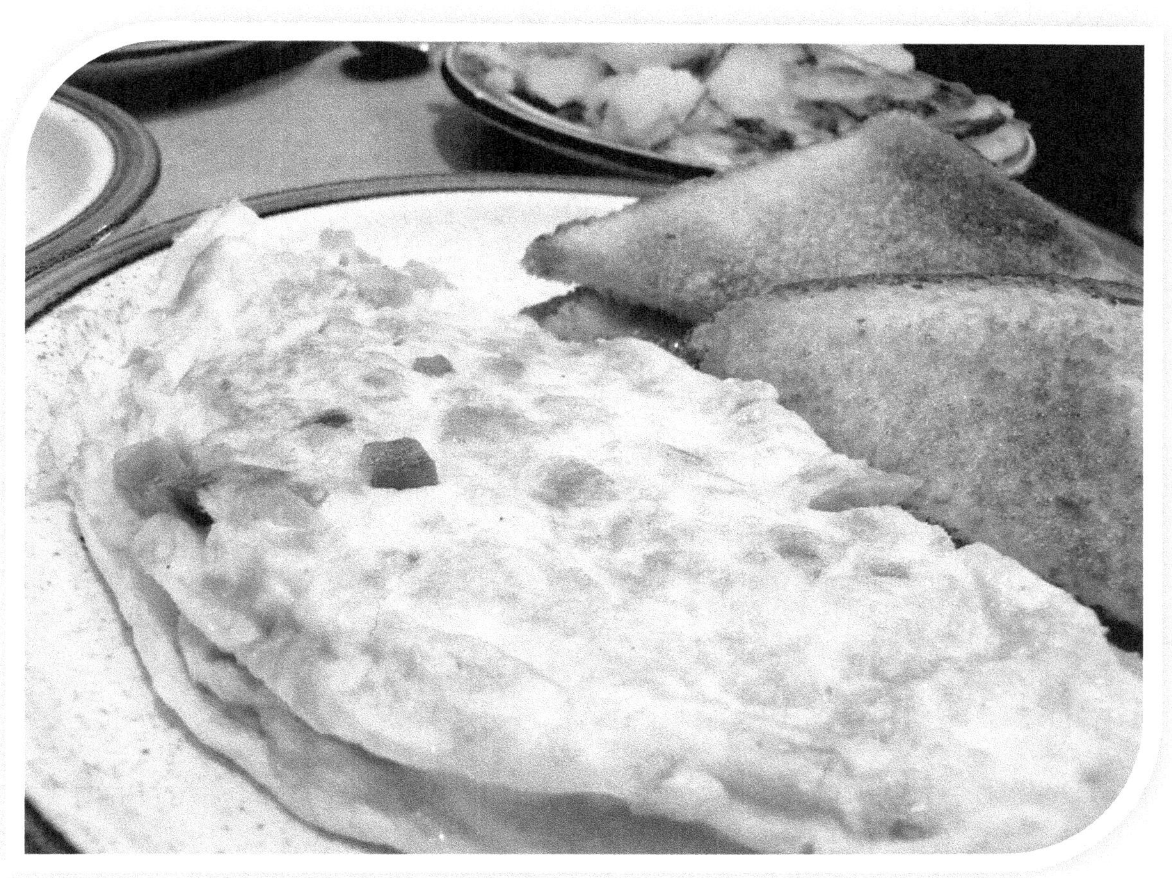

20. BAKED HADDOCK WITH CHEESY TOPPING

Ingredients

- For 4 servings
- 1 tbsp butter
- 1 shallot, sliced
- 1 lb haddock fillets
- 2 eggs, hard-boiled, chopped
- 3 tbsp hazelnut flour
- 2 cups sour cream
- 1 tbsp parsley, chopped
- ½ cup pork rinds, crushed
- 1 cup mozzarella cheese, grated
- Salt and black pepper to taste

Directions

Total Time: approx. 35 minutes

1. Melt butter in a saucepan over medium heat and sauté the shallot for 3 minutes.
2. Reduce the heat to low and stir in the hazelnut flour to form a roux.
3. Cook the roux until golden brown and stir in the sour cream until smooth.
4. Season to taste, and add parsley.
5. Arrange the haddock on a greased baking dish, sprinkle with the eggs, and spoon the sauce over.

6. In a bowl, mix the pork rinds with mozzarella, and spread the mixture over the sauce.

7. Bake in the oven for 20 minutes at 370 F until the top is golden and the sauce and cheese are bubbly. Serve warm.

Per serving:

- Cal 788
- Fat 57g
- Net Carbs 8.5g
- Protein 65g

VEGETABLE SIDES & DAIRY

21. ZUCCHINI & CHEESE CASSEROLE

Ingredients

For 4 servings

- 2 tbsp olive oil
- 1 tbsp salted butter, melted
- 3 large zucchinis, sliced
- ¼ cup grated mozzarella
- 2 /3 cup grated Parmesan
- 1 garlic clove, minced
- 1 tsp dried thyme

Directions

Total Time: approx. 25 minutes

1. Preheat oven to 350 F.
2. Pour zucchini in a bowl.
3. Add butter, olive oil, garlic, and thyme; toss to coat.
4. Spread onto a baking dish and sprinkle with the mozzarella and Parmesan cheeses.
5. Bake for 15 minutes. Serve warm.

Per serving:

- Cal 202
- Net Carbs 3g
- Fat 16g
- Protein 7.4g

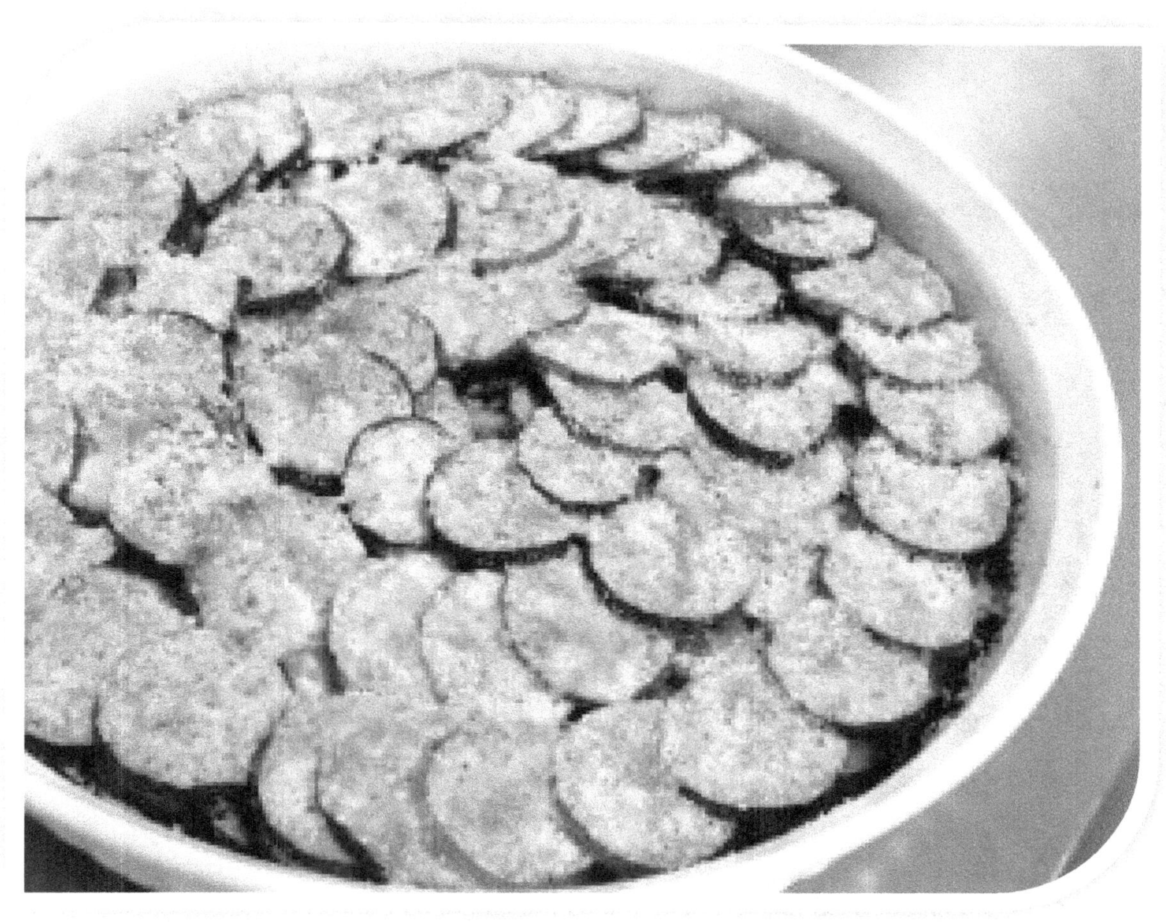

22. CRISPY AVOCADO WITH PARMESAN SAUCE

Ingredients

For 4 servings

- 1 tbsp olive oil
- 2 tbsp almond flour
- 1 ½ cups almond milk
- 5 tbsp melted butter
- 1 cup grated cheddar cheese
- 4 oz cream cheese, softened
- ¼ cup grated Parmesan
- 2 avocados, sliced
- ¼ tsp mustard powder
- ¼ tsp garlic powder
- 2 tbsp sriracha sauce
- Black pepper to taste

Directions

Total Time: approx. 20 minutes

1. Whisk 3 tbsps of butter with almond flour in a saucepan and cook until golden.
2. Whisk in almond milk, mustard powder, garlic powder, and black pepper.
3. Cook, whisking continuously until thickened, 2 minutes. Stir in the cheeses until they are melted; set aside .

4. In a bowl, toss avocado in the remaining butter and sriracha sauce.

5. Heat olive oil in a pan and cook avocado until golden, turning halfway, 4 minutes in total. P

6. late and pour the cheese sauce all over to serve.

Per serving:

- Cal 551
- Net Carbs 3.2g
- Fat 51g
- Protein 10g

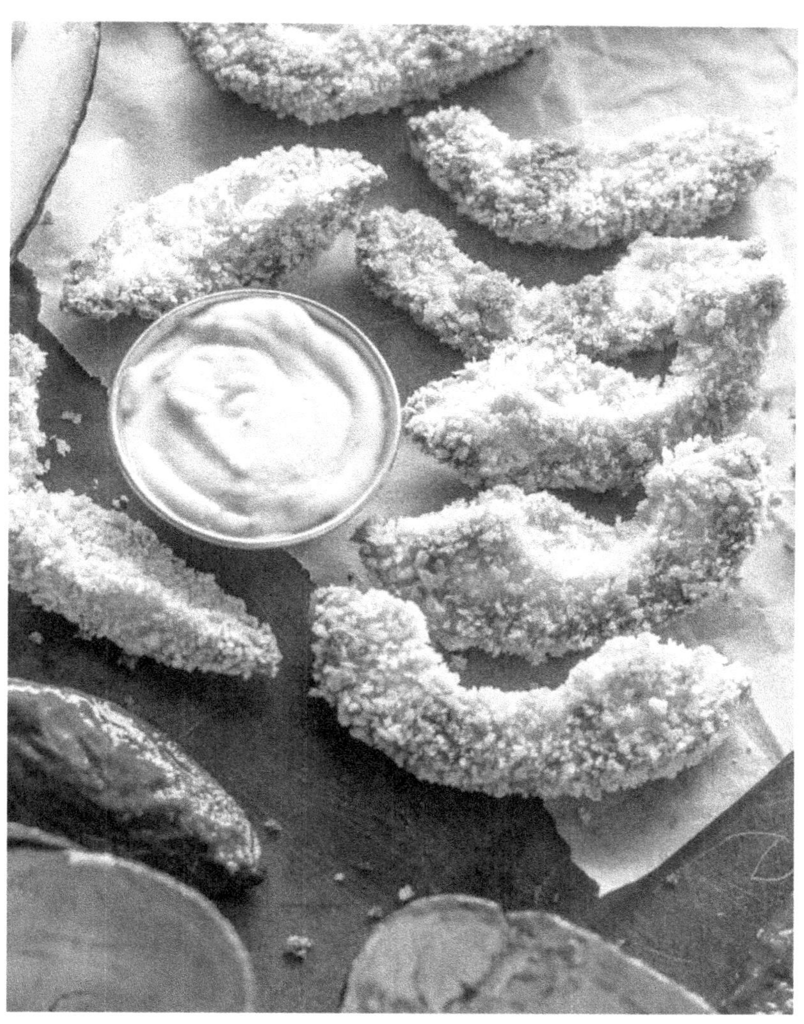

23. MUSHROOM & TOFU CAKES WITH CAULI MASH

Ingredients

For 4 servings
- 1 cup button mushrooms, chopped
- 1 lb tofu, pressed and cubed
- 2 garlic cloves, minced
- 2 small red onions, chopped
- 1 red bell pepper, chopped
- ½ cup golden flaxseed meal
- ½ almond milk
- 3 tbsp olive oil
- 2 cups tomato sauce
- 6 fresh basil leaves to garnish
- 1 lb cauliflower, cut into florets
- 2 tbsp butter
- ½ cup heavy cream
- ¼ cup grated Parmesan
- Salt and black pepper to taste

Directions

Total Time: approx. 65 minutes
1. Preheat oven to 360 F. Line a baking tray with parchment paper. In a bowl, add tofu, half of the garlic, half of the onion, mushrooms, salt, and pepper; mix to combine. Mold bite-size balls out of the mixture. Place flaxseed meal and almond milk each in a shallow dish. Dip each ball in almond milk and then in the flaxseed meal. Place on the baking sheet and bake for 10 minutes.
2. Heat 2 tbsp of olive oil in a saucepan and fry the tofu balls until golden brown on all sides, about 5-6 minutes; set aside. Heat the remaining oil in the same saucepan and sauté the remaining onion, remaining garlic, and bell pepper for 5 minutes. Pour in tomato sauce and cook for 10 minutes or until a stew forms. Add in tofu balls and simmer for 7 minutes.

3. In a pot, add cauliflower, 1 cup of water, and salt. Bring to a boil and cook for 10 minutes. Drain the cauliflower and pour it into a bowl. Add in butter, salt, and pepper; mash into a puree using a potato mash. Stir in heavy cream and Parmesan cheese until evenly combined. Spoon the mash into bowls, top with tofu balls and sauce, and garnish with basil leaves.

Per serving:
- Cal 692
- Net Carbs 5.6g
- Fat 28g
- Protein 19g

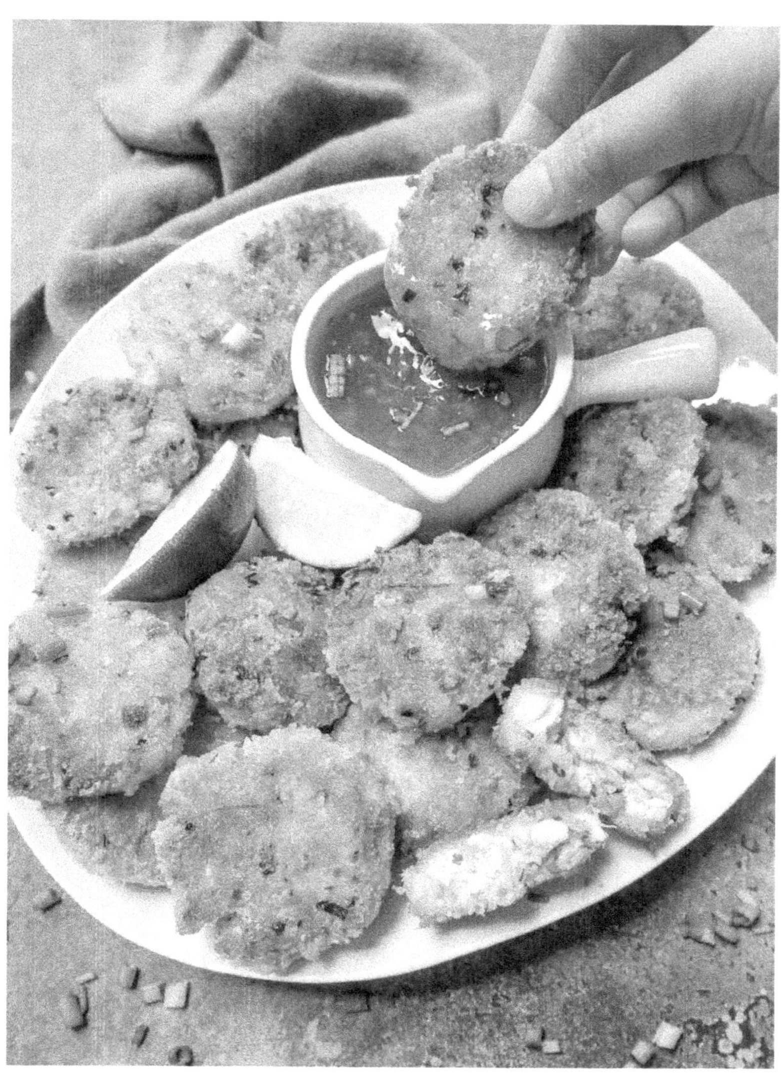

24. HOME-BAKE CHILI MACAROONS

Ingredients

For 4 servings

- 1 finger ginger root, peeled and pureed
- 3 egg whites
- ½ cup shredded coconut
- 1 tsp liquid stevia
- ¼ tsp chili powder
- ½ cup water
- Chili threads to garnish

Directions

Total Time: approx. 25 minutes

1. Line a baking sheet with parchment paper. In a heatproof bowl, whisk ginger, egg whites, shredded coconut, stevia, and chili powder.
2. In a pot over medium heat, bring to boil the water and place the heatproof bowl on the pot.
3. Continue whisking the mixture until it is glossy, about 4 minutes. Do not let the bowl touch the water or be too hot to cook the eggs.
4. Spoon the mixture into the piping bag and pipe out 40-50 little mounds on the lined baking sheet.
5. Bake the macaroons in the oven for 15 minutes at 350 F. Once they are ready, transfer them to a wire rack, garnish with chili threads to serve.

Per serving:

- Cal 110
- Fat 5.2g
- Net Carbs 1.4g
- Protein 8.3g

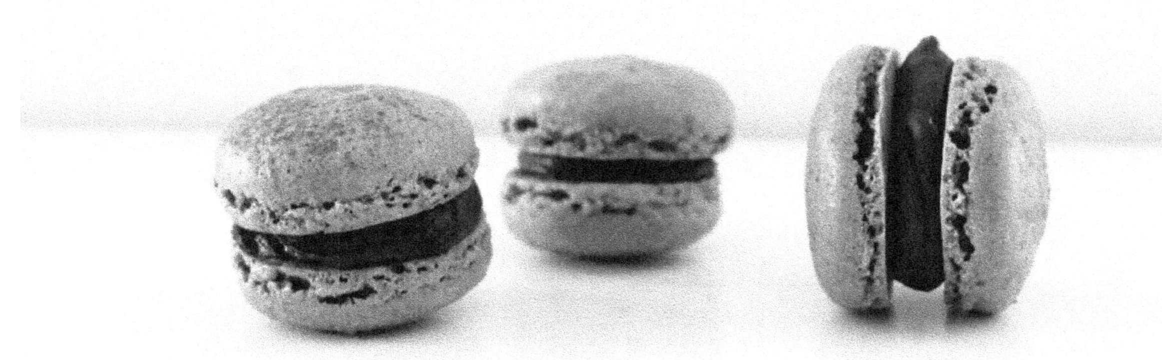

VEGAN

25. BASIL TOFU WITH CASHEW NUTS

Ingredients

For 4 servings

- 3 tsp olive oil
- 1 cup extra-firm tofu, cubed
- ¼ cup cashew nuts
- 1 ½ tbsp coconut aminos
- 3 tbsp vegetable broth 1 garlic clove, minced
- 1 tsp cayenne pepper
- ½ tsp turmeric powder
- Salt and black pepper to taste
- 2 tsp sunflower seeds
- 10 basil leaves, torn
- 1 tbsp balsamic vinegar

Directions

Total Time: approx. 25 minutes

1. Warm olive oil in a frying pan over medium heat.
2. Add in tofu and fry until golden, turning once, about 6 minutes.
3. Pour in the cashew nuts and cook for 2 minutes.
4. Stir in the remaining ingredients except for the balsamic vinegar and basil, set heat to medium-low, and cook for 5 more minutes.
5. Drizzle with the balsamic vinegar, season to taste, sprinkle with basil, and serve.

Per serving:

- Cal 245
- Fat 19g
- Net Carbs 5.5g
- Protein 12g

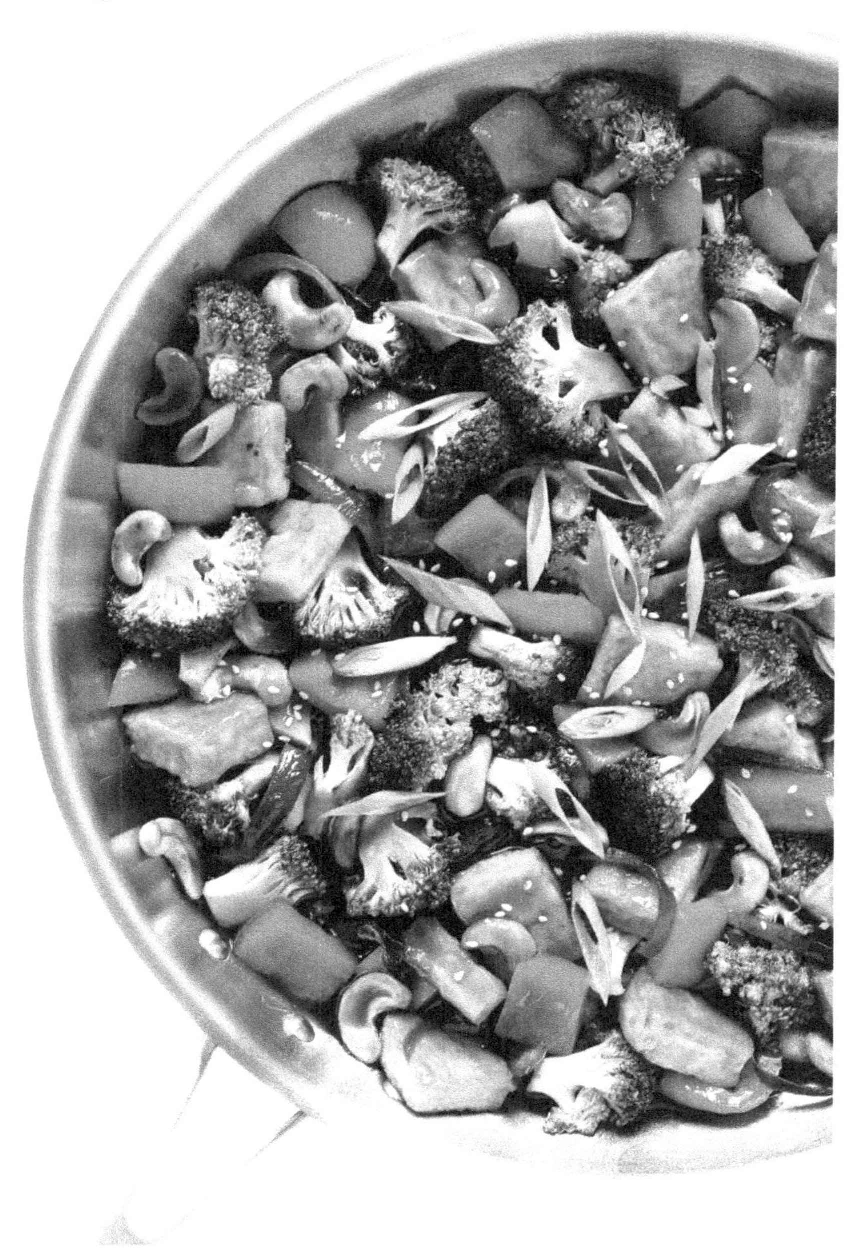

26. STEWED VEGETABLES

Ingredients

For 4 servings

- 2 tbsp olive oil
- 1 shallot, chopped
- 1 garlic clove, minced
- 1 tsp paprika
- 1 carrot, chopped
- 2 tomatoes, chopped
- 1 head cabbage, shredded
- 2 cups green beans, chopped
- 2 bell peppers, sliced
- Salt and black pepper to taste
- 2 tbsp parsley, chopped
- 1 cup vegetable broth

Directions

Total Time: approx. 45 minutes

1. Warm the olive oil in a saucepan over medium heat and sauté onion and garlic until fragrant, 2 minutes.
2. Stir in bell peppers, carrot, cabbage, green beans, paprika, salt, and pepper for 4-5 minutes.
3. Add vegetable broth and tomatoes and cook on low heat for 25 minutes to soften.
4. Serve sprinkled with parsley.

Per serving:

- Cal 310
- Fat 26.4g
- Net Carbs 6g
- Protein 8g

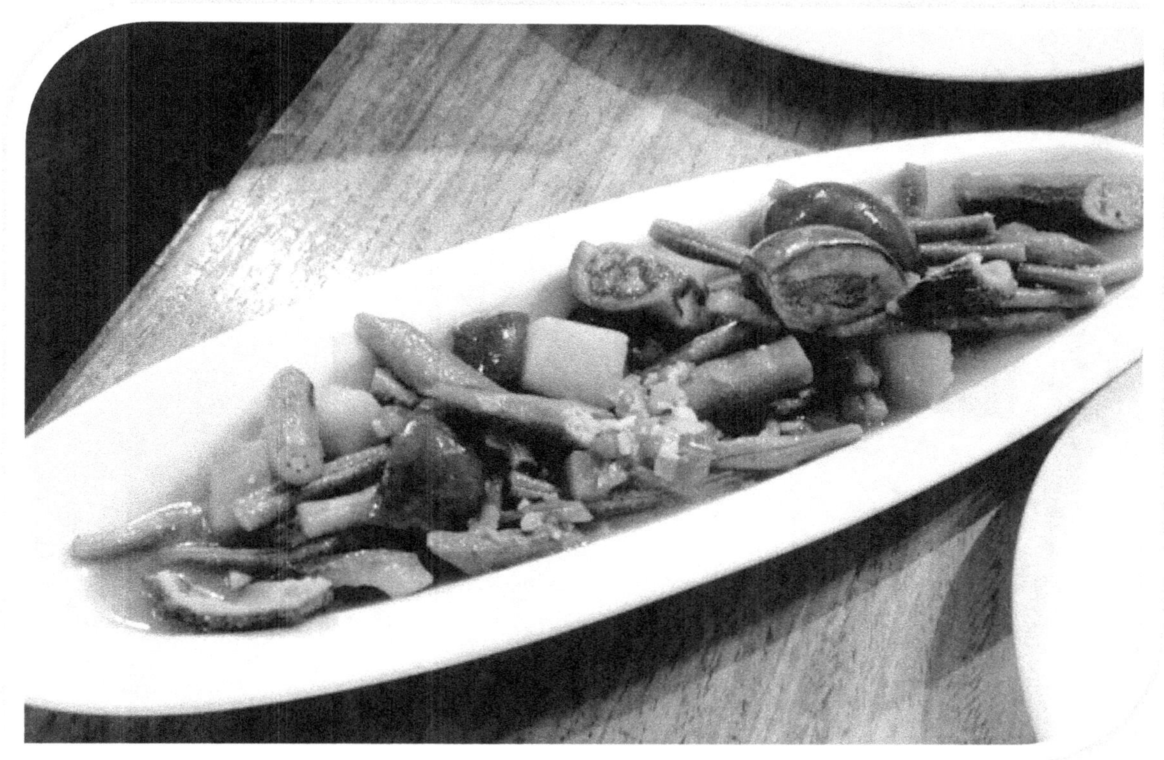

SNACKS & APPETIZERS

27. CHICKEN RANCH PIZZA WITH BACON & BASIL

Ingredients

For 4 servings

- 1 tbsp butter
- 2 chicken breasts
- 3 cups shredded mozzarella
- 3 tbsp cream cheese, softened
- ¾ cup almond flour 2 tbsp almond meal
- ¼ cup half and half
- 1 tbsp dry Ranch seasoning
- 3 bacon slices, chopped
- 6 fresh basil leaves

Directions

Total Time: approx. 50 minutes

1. Preheat oven to 390 F. Line a pizza pan with parchment paper. Microwave 2 cups of mozzarella cheese and 2 tbsp of the cream cheese for 30 seconds.

2. Mix in almond flour and almond meal. Spread the "dough" on the pan and bake for 15 minutes.

3. In a bowl, mix butter, remaining cream cheese, half and half, and ranch mix; set aside.

4. Heat a grill pan and cook the bacon for 5 minutes; set aside. Grill the chicken in the pan on both sides for 10 minutes.

5. Remove to a plate, allow cooling, and cut into thin slices. Spread the ranch sauce on the pizza crust, followed by the chicken and bacon, and then the remaining mozzarella and basil.

6. Bake for 5 minutes.

Per serving:

- Cal 531
- Net Carbs 4g
- Fats 32g
- Protein 62g

-

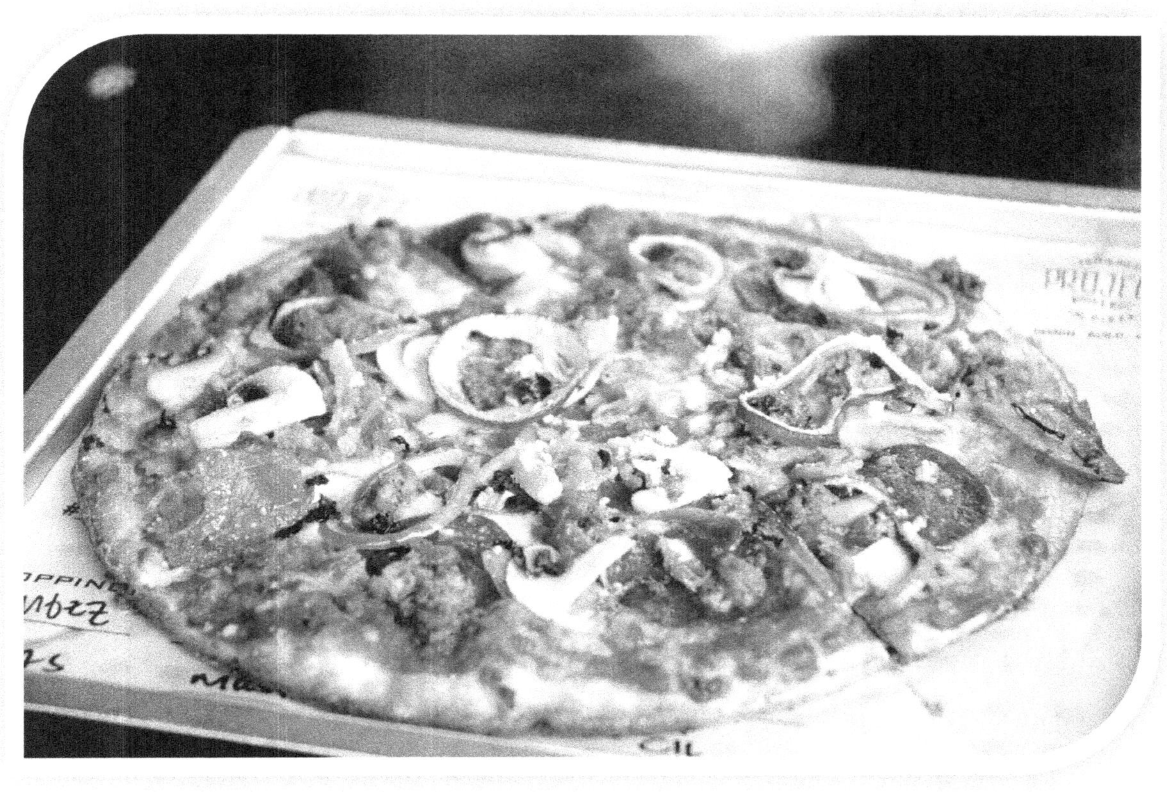

28. EGGPLANT & BACON GRATIN

Ingredients

for 4 servings

- 3 large eggplants, sliced
- 6 bacon slices, chopped
- ½ cup shredded Parmesan
- ½ cup crumbled feta cheese
- 1 tbsp dried oregano
- ¾ cup heavy cream
- 2 tbsp chopped parsley
- Salt and black pepper to taste

Directions

Total Time: approx. 45 minutes

1. Preheat oven to 380 F. Put bacon in a skillet and fry over medium heat until brown and crispy, 6 minutes.
2. Transfer to a plate. Arrange half of the eggplants in a greased baking sheet and season with oregano, parsley, salt, and pepper. Scatter half of bacon and half of feta cheese on top and repeat the remaining ingredients' layering process.
3. In a bowl, combine heavy cream with half of the Parmesan cheese, and spread on top of the layered ingredients.
4. Sprinkle with the remaining Parmesan.
5. Bake until the cream is bubbly, 20 minutes. Serve.

Per serving:

- Cal 429
- Net Carbs 1.7g
- Fat 30g
- Protein 16g

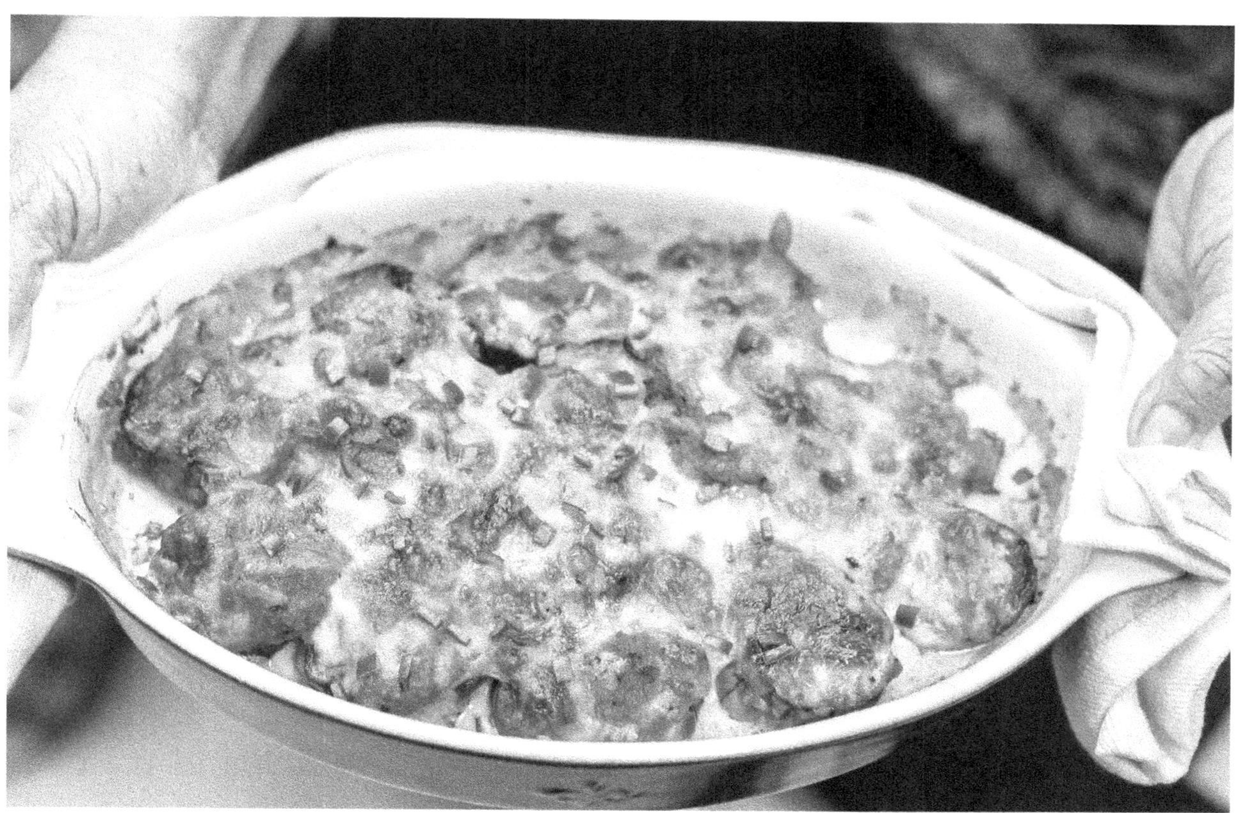

29. CREAMY CELERIAC & BACON BAKE

Ingredients

For 4 servings

- 3 tbsp butter
- 6 bacon slices, chopped
- 3 garlic cloves, minced
- 3 tbsp almond flour
- 2 cups coconut cream
- 1 cup chicken broth
- 1 lb celeriac, peeled and sliced
- 2 cups shredded cheddar
- ¼ cup chopped scallions
- Salt and black pepper to taste

Directions

Total Time: approx. 50 minutes

1. Preheat oven to 380 F. Add bacon to a skillet and fry over medium heat until brown and crispy. Spoon onto a plate.
2. Melt butter in the same skillet and sauté garlic for 1 minute. Mix in almond flour and cook for another minute.
3. Whisk in coconut cream, chicken broth, salt, and pepper. Simmer for 5 minutes.
4. Spread a layer of the sauce in a greased casserole dish and arrange a celeriac layer on top.
5. Cover with more sauce, top with some bacon and cheddar cheese, and scatter scallions on top.

6. Repeat the layering process until the ingredients are exhausted. Bake for 35 minutes.

7. Let rest for a few minutes and serve.

Per serving:

- Cal 979
- Net Carbs 20g
- Fat 79g
- Protein 30g

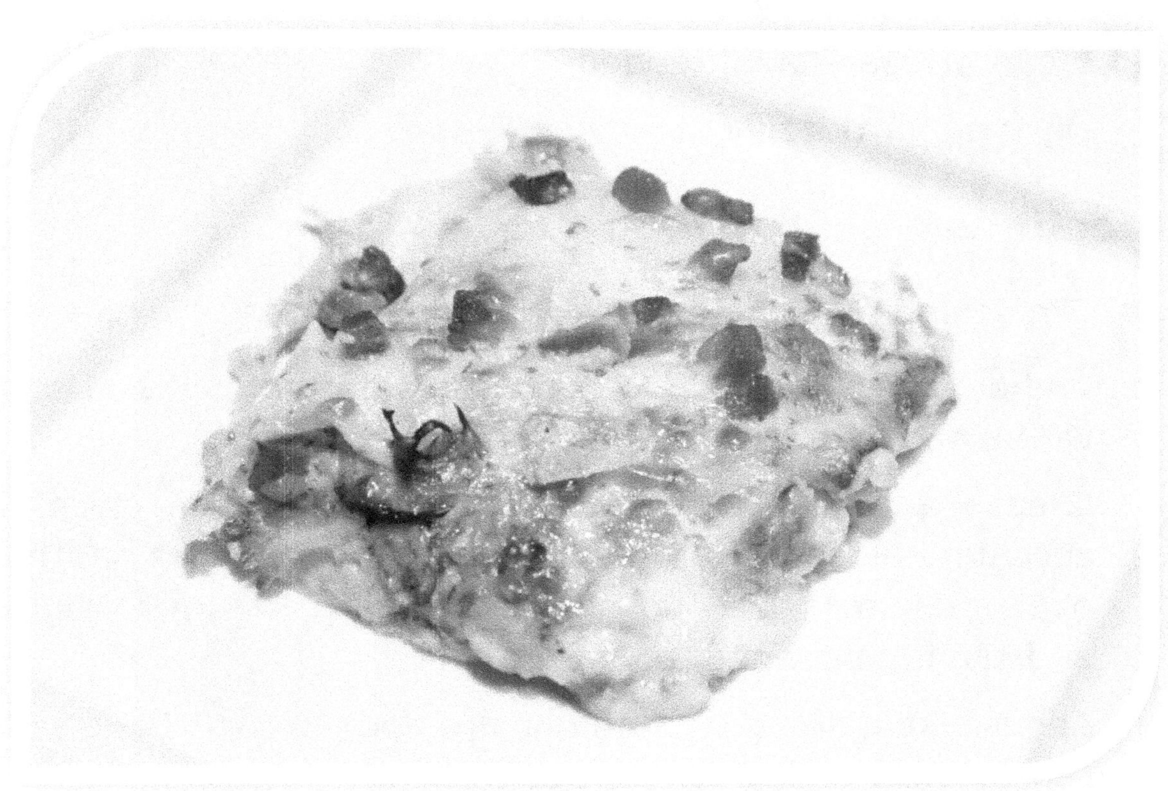

30. KALE & CHEESE STUFFED ZUCCHINI

Ingredients

For 2 servings

- 1 zucchini, halved
- 4 tbsp butter
- 2 garlic cloves, minced
- 1 ½ oz baby kale
- Salt and black pepper to taste
- 2 tbsp tomato sauce
- 1 cup mozzarella, shredded
- Olive oil for drizzling

Directions

Total Time: approx. 40 minutes

1. Preheat oven to 375 F. Scoop out the pulp of the zucchini with a spoon into a plate; keep the flesh.

2. Grease a baking sheet with cooking spray and place the zucchini halves on top. Put the butter in a skillet and melt over medium heat. Add and sauté the garlic until fragrant and slightly browned, about 4 minutes.

3. Add the kale and the zucchini pulp. Cook until the kale wilts; season with salt and black pepper.

4. Spoon the tomato sauce into the zucchini halves and spread to coat the bottom evenly. Spoon the kale mixture into the zucchinis and sprinkle with the mozzarella cheese. Bake in the oven for 20-25 minutes or until the cheese has a

beautiful golden color. Plate the zucchinis when ready, drizzle with olive oil, and season with salt and black pepper.

Per serving:

- Cal 345
- Fat 25g
- Net Carbs 6.9g
- Protein 2g

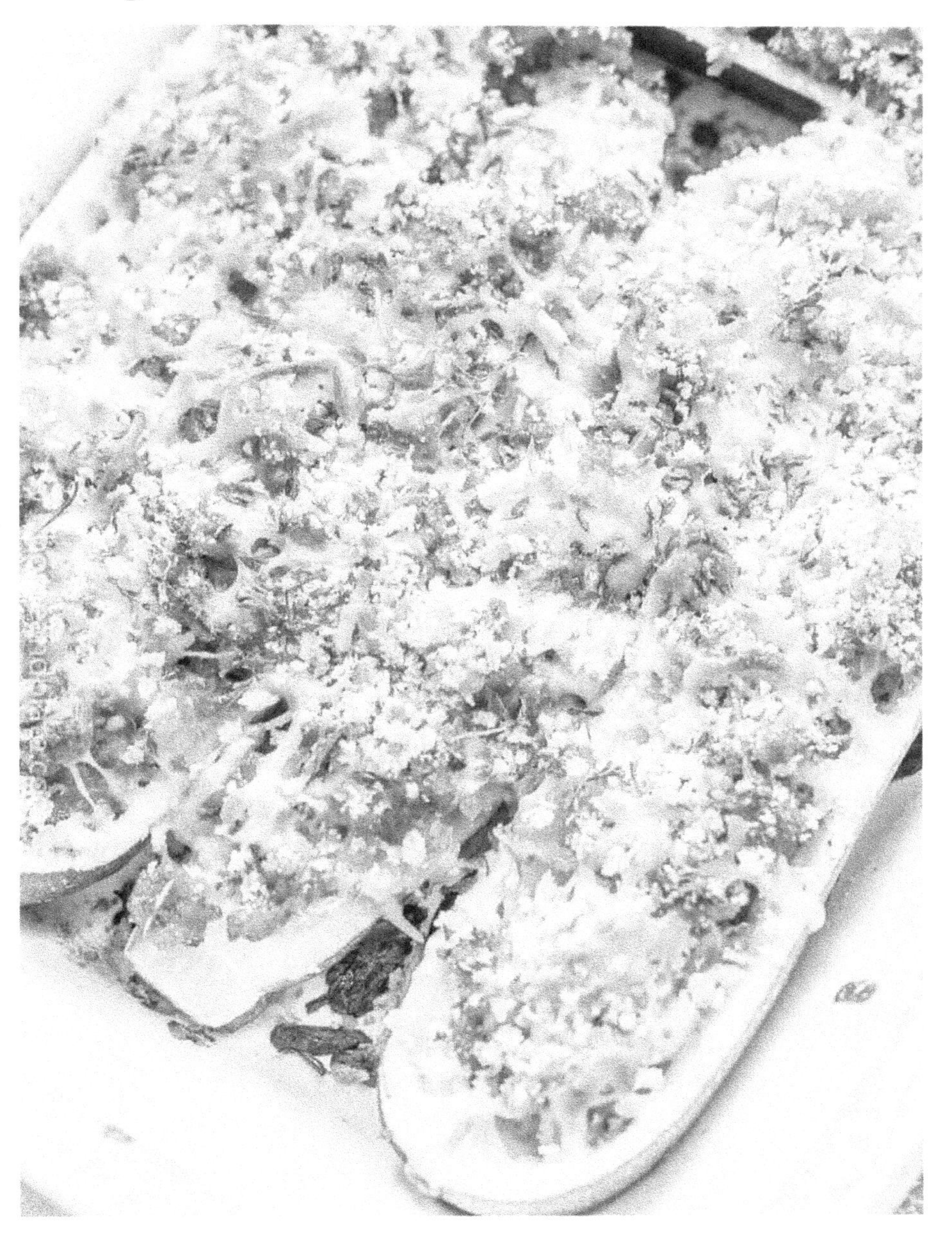

31. MINI SAUSAGES WITH SWEET MUSTARD SAUCE

Ingredients

For 4 servings

- 2b mini smoked sausages
- 3tbsp almond flour
- 2 tsp mustard powder
- ¼ cup lemon juice
- ¼ cup white wine vinegar
- 1 cup Swerve brown sugar
- 1 tsp tamari sauce

Directions

Total Time: approx. 15 minutes

1. In a pot, combine Swerve brown sugar, almond flour, and mustard.
2. Gradually stir in lemon juice, vinegar, and tamari sauce. Bring to a boil over medium heat while stirring until thickened, 2 minutes.
3. Mix in sausages until adequately coated. Cook them for 5 minutes. Serve.

Per serving:

- Cal 751
- Net Carbs 7.2g
- Fat 45g; Protein 24g

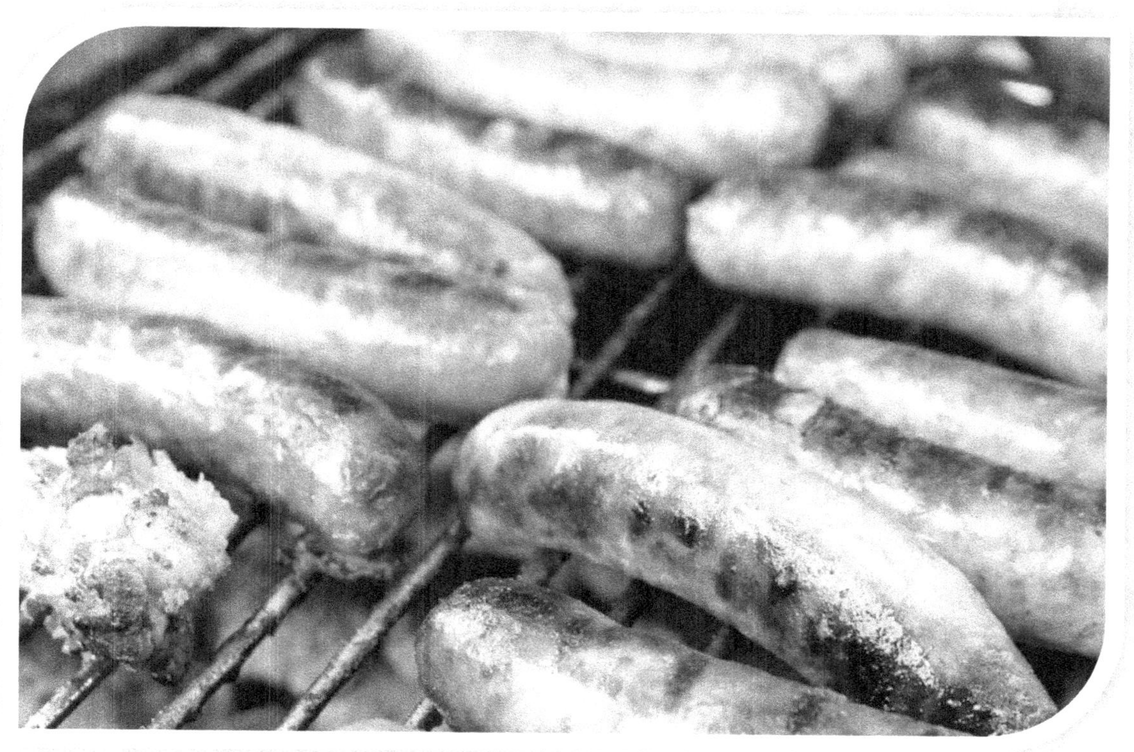

32. PANCETTA & BROCCOLI ROAST

Ingredients

For 4 servings

- 6 pancetta slices, chopped
- 1 lb broccoli rabe, halved
- 2 bsp olive oil
- ¼ tsp red chili flakes

Directions

Total Time: approx. 40 minutes

1. Preheat oven to 420 F. Place broccoli rabe in a greased baking sheet and top with pancetta.
2. Drizzle with olive oil, season to taste, and sprinkle with chili flakes.
3. Roast for 30 minutes. Serve warm and enjoy!

Per serving:

- Cal 130
- Net Carbs 0.2g
- Fat 10g
- Protein 6.8g

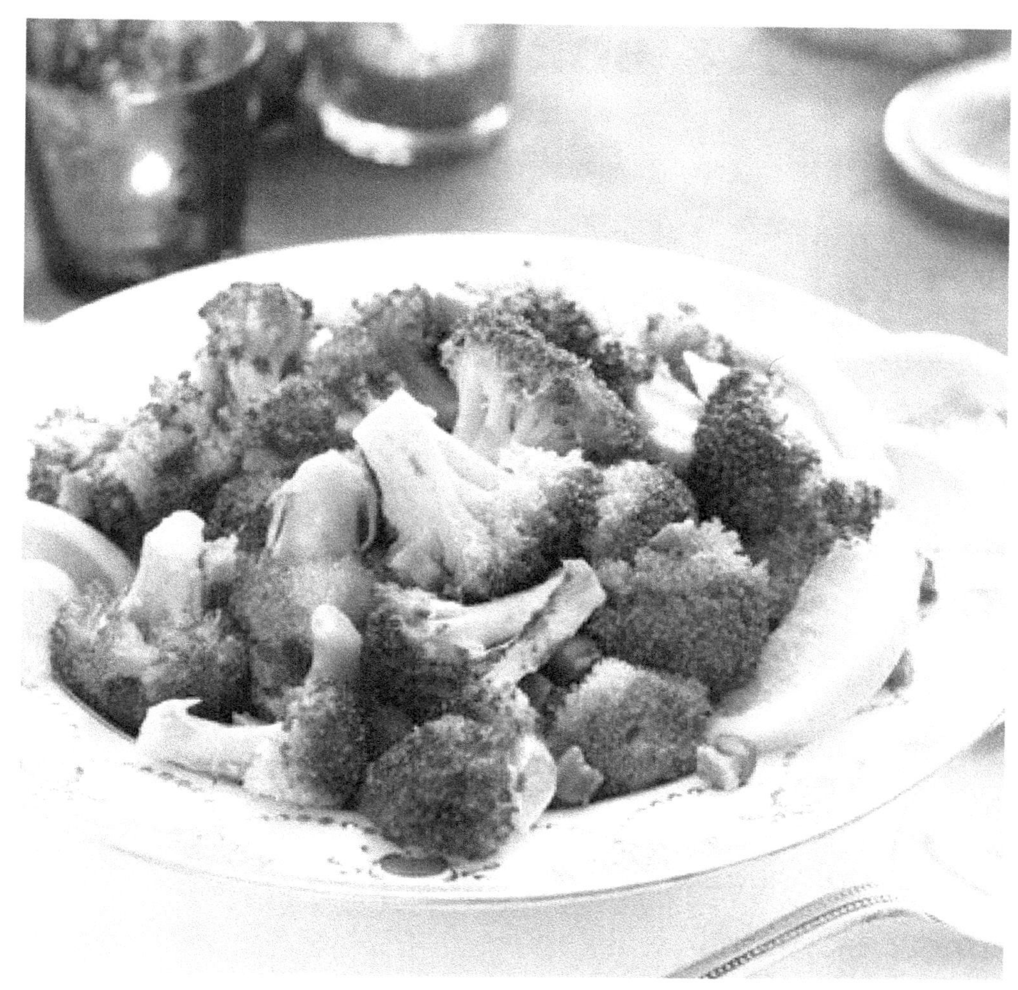

33. FETA & BOK CHOY STIR-FRY

Ingredients

for 2 servings

- 2 ½ cups baby bok choy, quartered lengthwise
- 5 oz butter
- 2 cups feta cheese, crumbled
- Salt and black pepper to taste
- 1 tsp garlic powder 1 tsp onion powder
- 1 tbsp plain vinegar
- 2 garlic cloves, minced
- 1 tsp chili flakes
- 3 green onions, sliced
- 1 tbsp sesame oil

Directions

Total Time: approx. 25 minutes

1. Melt half of the butter in a wok over medium heat, add the bok choy, and stir-fry until softened.
2. Season with salt, black pepper, garlic powder, onion powder, and plain vinegar.
3. Sauté for 2 minutes and then spoon the bok choy into a bowl; set aside.
4. Melt the remaining butter in the wok.
5. Sauté the garlic and chili flakes until fragrant.
6. Add green onions, feta, and bok choy, heat for 2 minutes, and add the sesame oil.

7. Serve with steamed cauli rice.

Per serving:

- Cal 641
- Fat 53g
- Net Carbs 7.8g
- Protein 31g

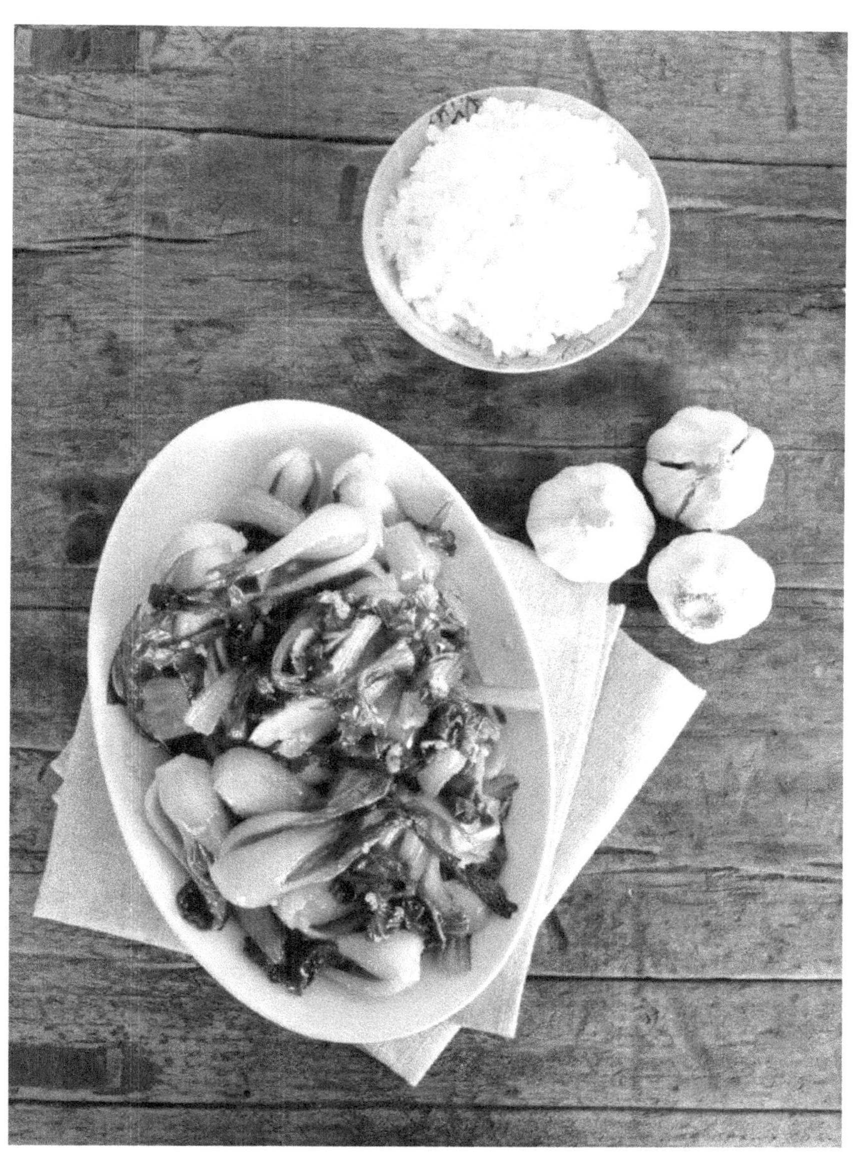

SMOOTHIES
&
BEVERAGES

34. STRAWBERRY LEMONADE WITH BASIL

Ingredients

For 4 servings

- 1 /3 cup fresh mint, reserve some for garnishing
- 12 strawberries
- ¼ cup fresh lemon juice
- ½ cup erythritol
- Crushed Ice
- Halved strawberries to garnish
- Basil leaves to garnish

Directions

Total Time: approx. 10 minutes

1. Add some ice into 2 serving glasses and set aside.
2. In a pitcher of a blender, add 2 cups of water, strawberries, lemon juice, mint, and erythritol.
3. Process the ingredients for 30 seconds.
4. The mixture should be pink and the mint finely chopped.
5. Adjust the taste and divide between the ice glasses.
6. Drop 2 strawberry halves and basil leaves in each glass and serve immediately.

Per serving:

- Cal 36

- Fat 0.7g
- Net Carbs 5.1g
- Protein 1.5g

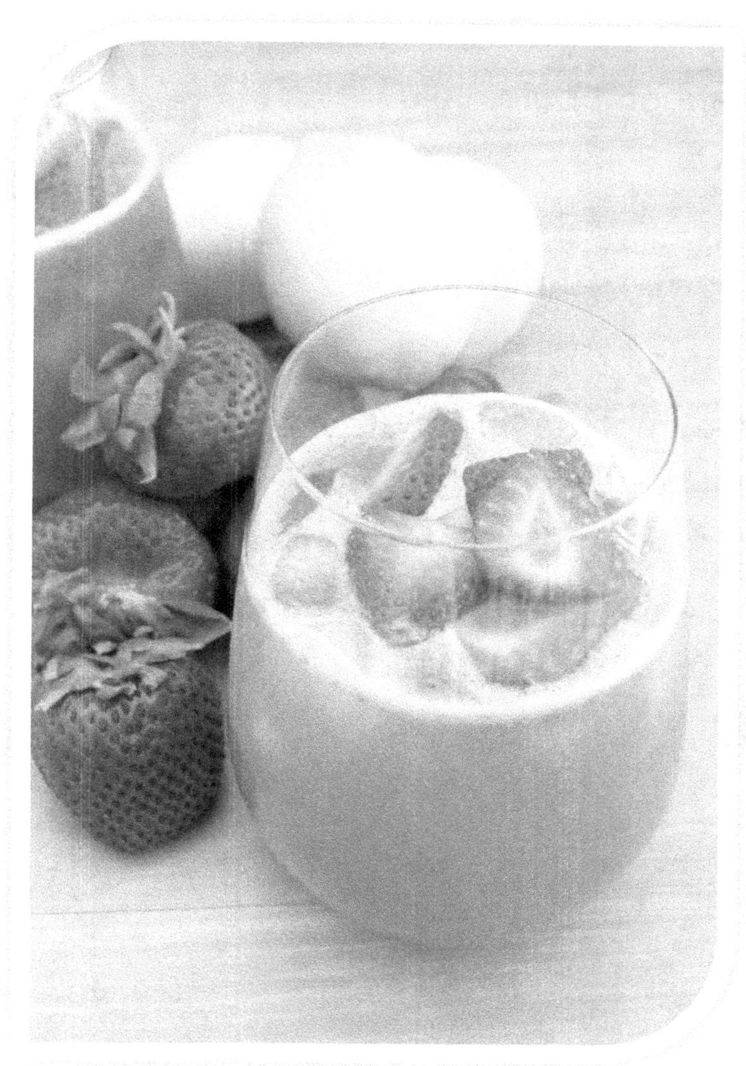

35. COLD MATCHA LATTE

Ingredients

For 2 servings

- 2 tsp matcha green tea powder
- 1 /3 cup almond milk, cold

Directions

Total Time: approx. 10 minutes

1. Warm 2 cups of water in your microwave.
2. Divide the matcha green tea powder between them and whisk well until there are no lumps.
3. Stir in cold almond milk for an iced latte. Serve and enjoy!
4. Warm the milk in a small saucepan and pour into the mug until nearly full.
5. Use cold milk for an iced latte.

Per serving:

- Cal 95
- Fat 9.5g
- Net Carbs 1.3g
- Protein 1.9g

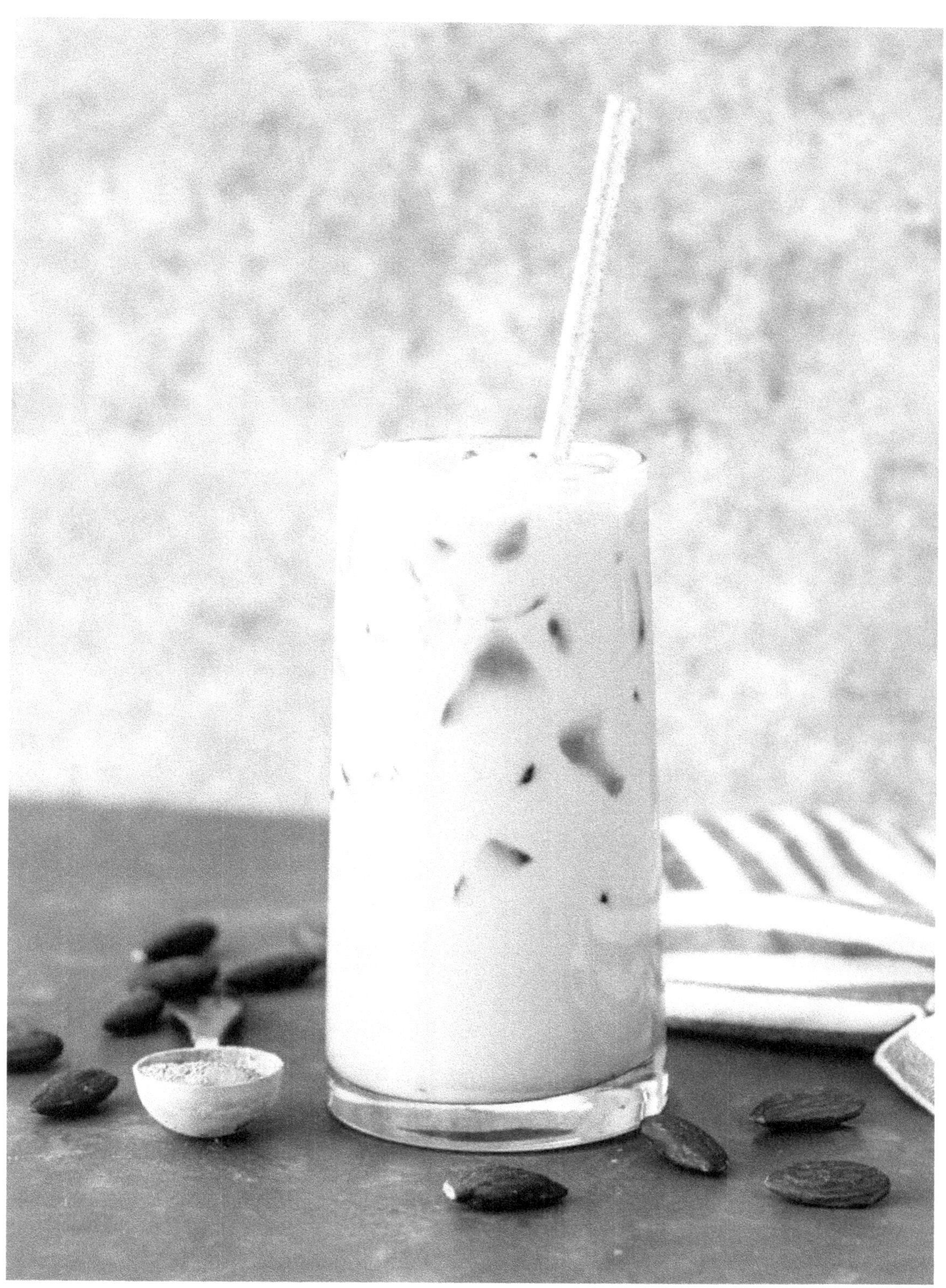

SWEETS & DESSERTS

36. CLASSIC LEMON CURD TARTS

Ingredients

For 4 servings

For the crust

- ¼ cup Swerve confectioner's sugar
- 1 large egg
- ¼ cup butter, melted
- 1 ½ cups almond flour
- ½ tsp salt

For the filling

- ½ cup Swerve confectioner's sugar
- 4 tbsp salted butter
- ½ lemon, zested and juiced
- 3 large eggs

Directions

Total Time: approx. 30 min + chilling time

1. Preheat oven to 360 F. Lightly grease 4 mini tart tins with cooking spray.
2. In a food processor, blend almond flour, Swerve sugar, salt, butter, and egg.
3. Divide and spread the dough on the tins.

4. Bake for 15 minutes. For the filling, melt butter in a saucepan over medium heat, take off the heat and quickly mix in Swerve sugar, lemon zest, and lemon juice until smooth.

5. Whisk in eggs and return the saucepan to low heat. Cook with continuous stirring until thick.

6. Pour the filling into the crust, gently tap on a flat surface to release air bubbles, and chill in the refrigerator.

Per serving:

- Cal 209
- Net Carbs 2g
- Fat 19g
- Protein 7g

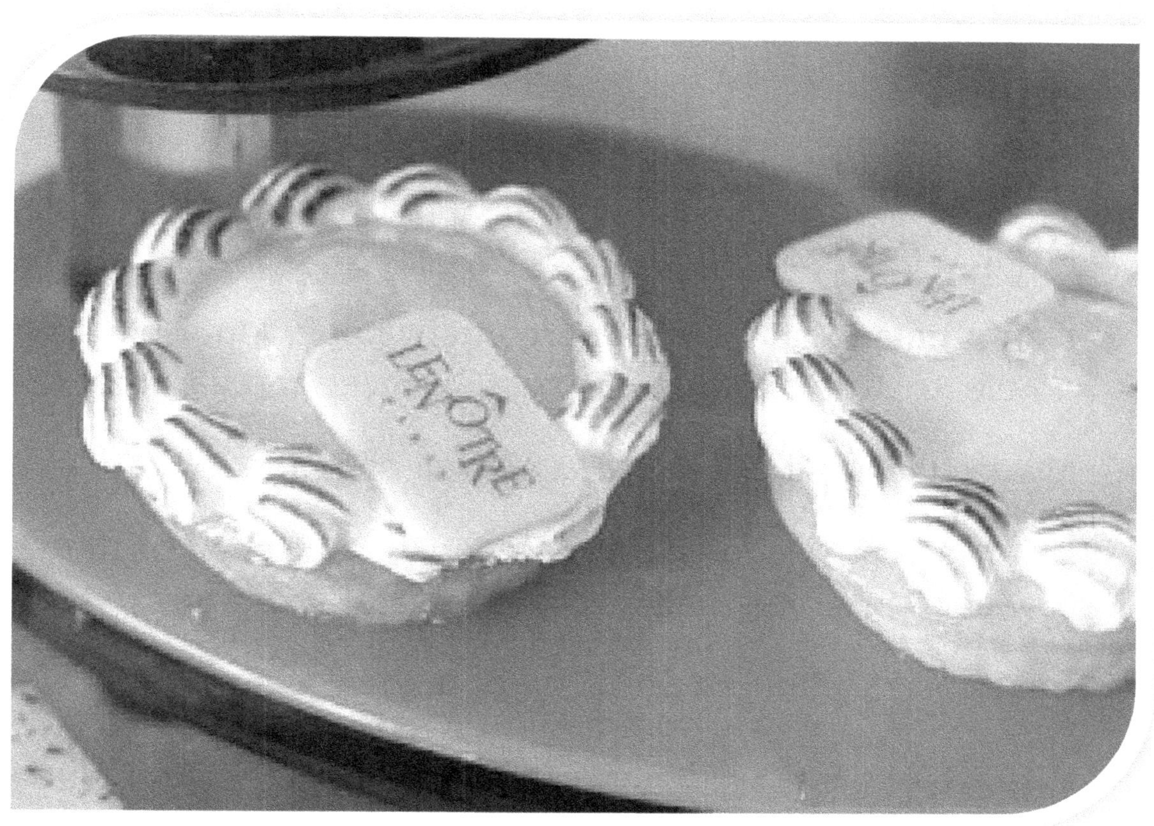

37. CHOCOLATE & CARAMEL SHORTBREAD COOKIES

Ingredients

For 6 servings

- ¼ cup sugar- free caramel sauce
- 1 cup chopped dark chocolate
- 2 cups butter, softened
- 1 ½ cups Swerve brown sugar
- 3 cups almond flour
- Sea salt flakes

Directions

Total Time: approx. 30 minutes

1. Preheat oven to 360 F.
2. Line a baking sheet with parchment paper. In a bowl, using an electric mixer, whisk butter, Swerve, and caramel sauce.
3. Mix in flour and chocolate until well combined.
4. Using a scoop, spoon 1 ½ tbsp of the batter onto the sheet at 2-inch intervals and sprinkle salt flakes on top.
5. Bake for 15 minutes until lightly golden.

Per serving:

- Cal 409

- Net Carbs 0.6g
- Fat 43g
- Protein 4.9g

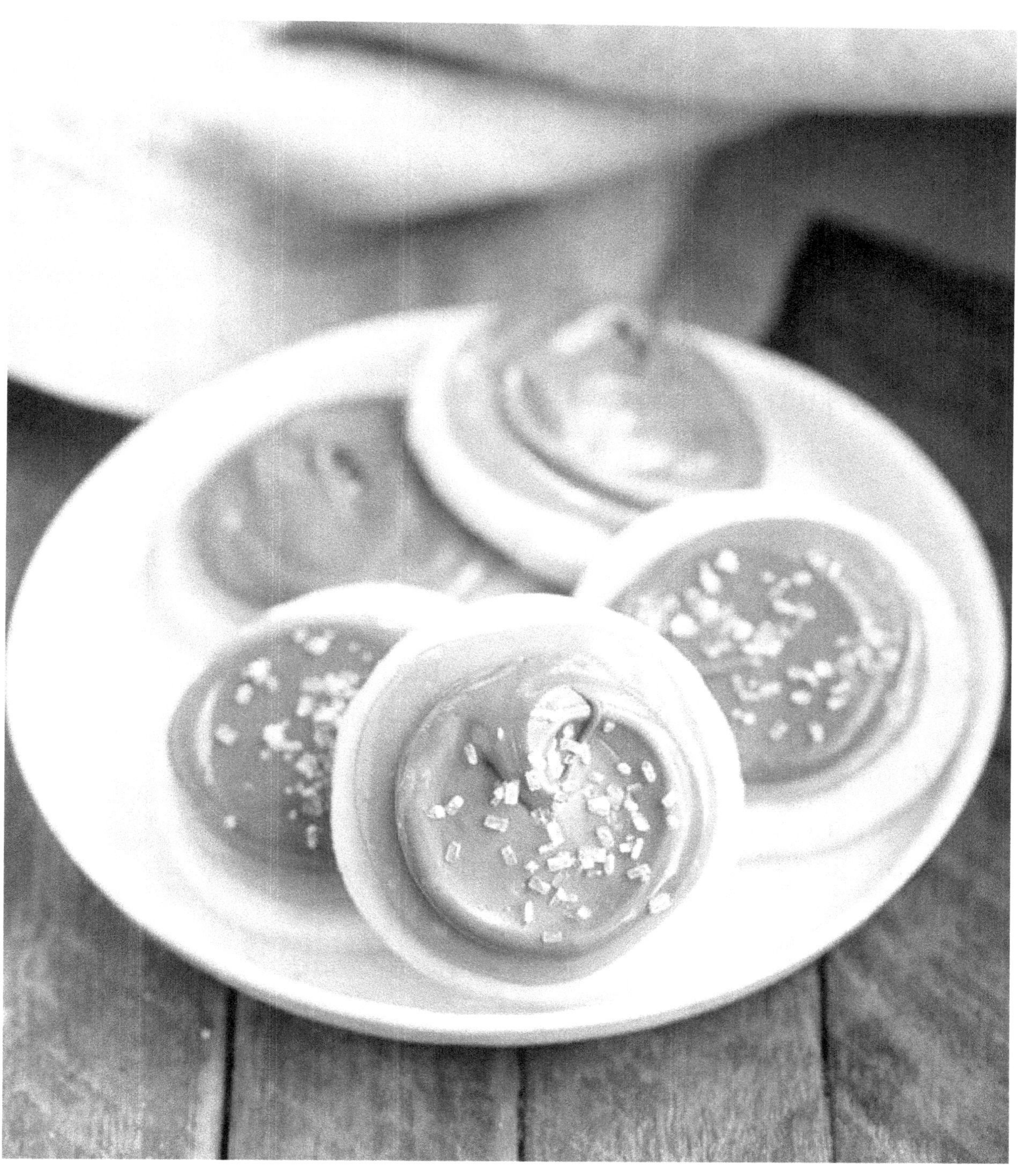

38. VALENTINE'S DAY COOKIES

Ingredients

For 4 servings

- 2 cups almond flour + extra for dusting
- ½ cup unsweetened dark chocolate
- ½ lemon, zested
- 1 cup unsalted butter, softened
- 2 /3 cup Swerve sugar
- 1 large egg, beaten
- 2 tsp vanilla extract
- 2 tbsp chopped pistachios

Directions

Total Time: approx. 30 min + chilling time

1. Preheat oven to 350 F. Add the butter and Swerve sugar to a bowl; beat with an electric whisk until smooth and creamy.

2. Whisk in the egg until combined.

3. Mix in the vanilla extract, lemon zest, and almond flour until a soft dough forms. Wrap the dough in plastic wrap and chill for 10 minutes.

4. Dust a chopping board with some almond flour. Unwrap the dough and roll out on the chopping board to 2-inch thickness.

5. Using a cookie cutter, cut out as many biscuits as you can get while rerolling the trimming and making more biscuits.

6. Arrange the biscuits on the parchment paper-lined baking sheet and bake for 12 to 15 minutes or until crisp at the edges and pale golden.

7. Remove and transfer to a wire rack to cool completely when ready. In two separate bowls, melt the chocolate in your microwave.

8. Dip one side of each biscuit in the dark chocolate. Garnish the dark chocolate's side with the pistachios and allow cooling on the wire rack.

Per serving:

- Cal 476
- Fat 43.5g
- Net Carbs 5g
- Protein 4.5g

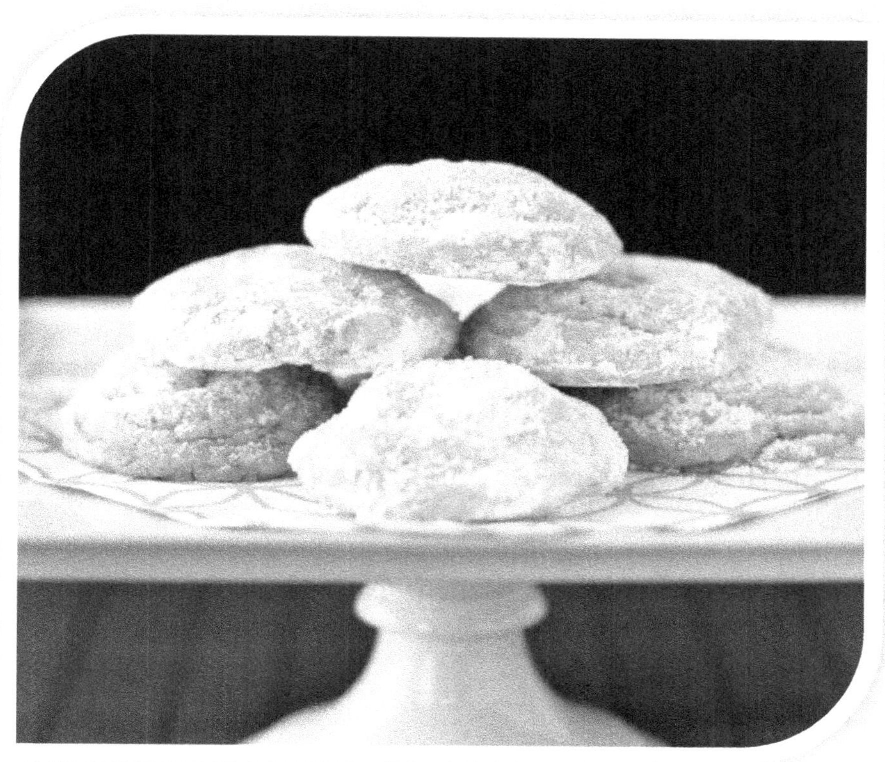

39. VANILLA CHEESECAKE COOKIES

Ingredients

For 4 servings

- 1 large egg
- 2 tsp vanilla extract
- ¼ cup softened butter
- 2 oz softened cream cheese
- 1 /3 cup xylitol
- ¼ tsp salt
- 1 tbsp sour cream
- 3 cups blanched almond flour

Directions

Total Time: approx. 25 minutes

1. Preheat oven to 360 F.
2. Line a baking sheet with parchment paper. Using an electric mixer, whisk butter, cream cheese, and xylitol in a bowl until fluffy and light in color.
3. Beat in egg, vanilla, salt, and sour cream until smooth.
4. Add in flour and mix until soft batter forms. With a cookie scoop, arrange 1 ½ tbsp of batter onto the sheet at 2-inch intervals.
5. Bake for 15 minutes until lightly golden.
6. Let cool before serving.

Per serving:

- Cal 180
- Net Carbs 1.3g
- Fat 17g
- Protein 2.9g

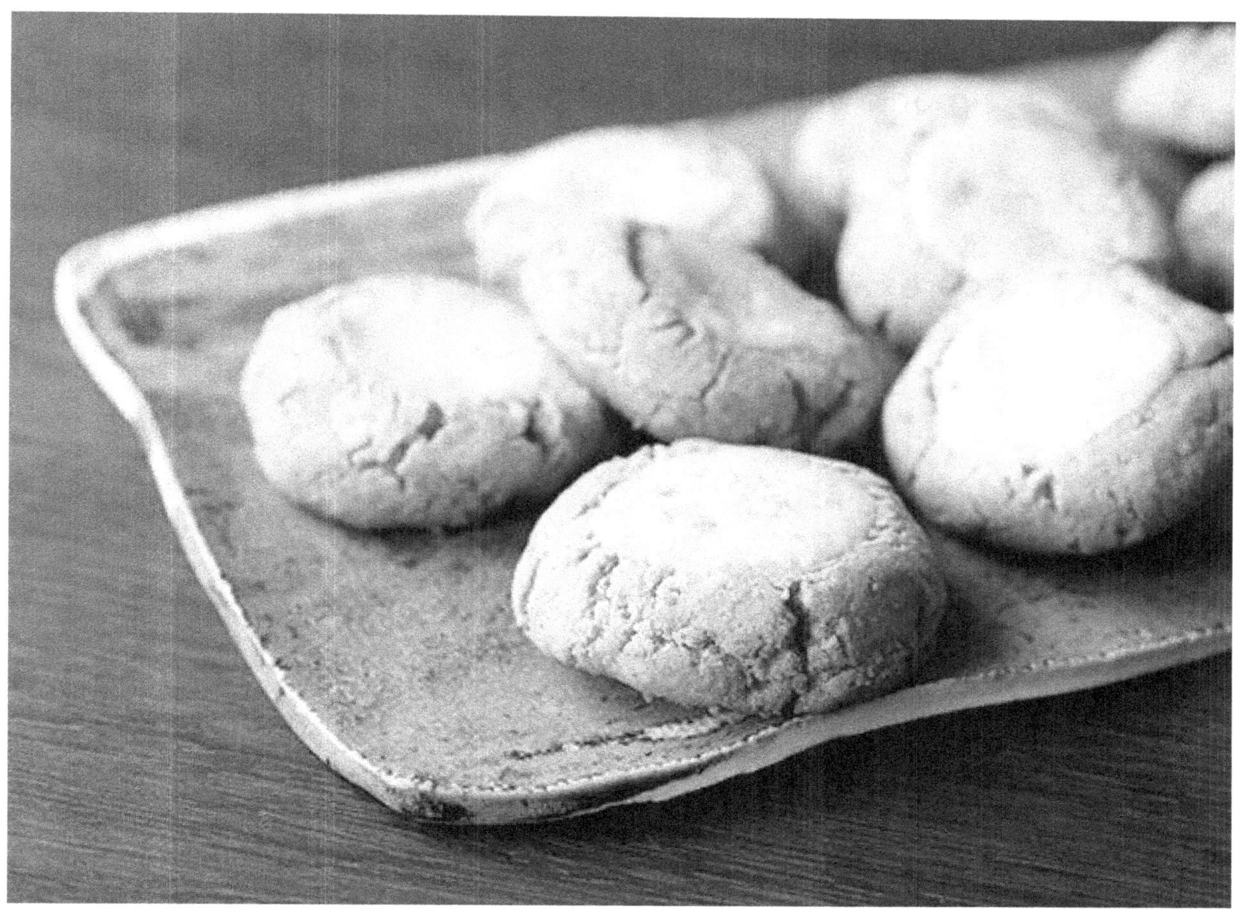

40. SUNDAY CHOCOLATE COOKIES

Ingredients

For 4 servings

- 2 cups unsweetened dark chocolate chips
- 7 oz butter, softened
- 2 cups Swerve brown sugar
- 3 eggs
- 2 cups almond flour

Directions

Total Time: approx. 30 minutes

1. Line a baking sheet with parchment paper.
2. Preheat oven to 330 F.
3. In a bowl with a hand mixer, whisk the butter and Swerve sugar for 3 minutes or until light and fluffy.
4. Add the eggs one at a time and scrape the sides as you whisk.
5. Mix in almond flour at low speed until well combined.
6. Fold in chocolate chips.
7. Scoop 3 tablespoons each on the baking sheet, creating spaces between each mound, and bake for 15 minutes to swell and harden.
8. Remove, cool, and serve.

Per serving:

- Cal 293

- Fat 24.5g

- Net Carbs 7.3g

- Protein 6g

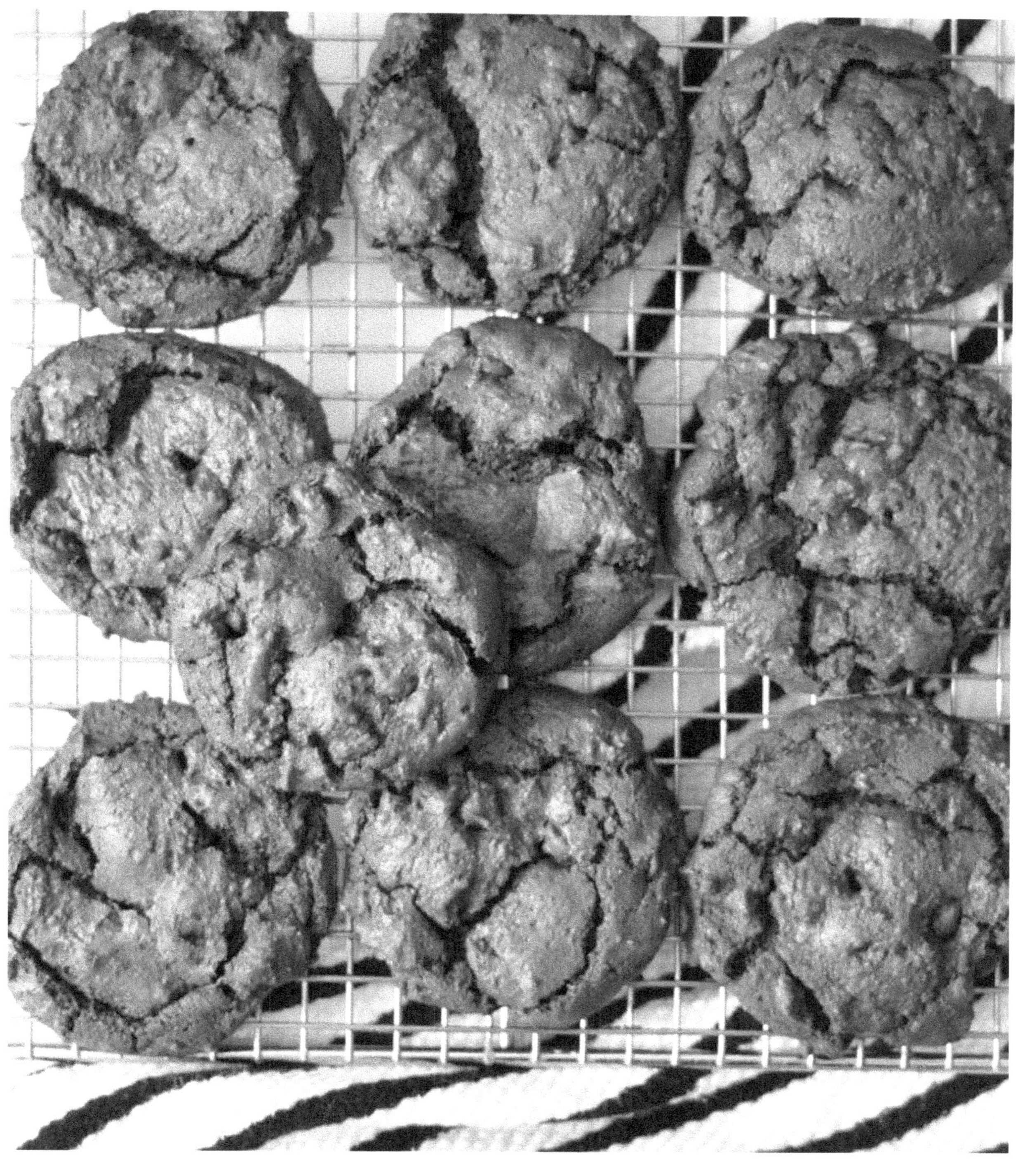

41. ALMOND COOKIES

Ingredients

For 4 servings

- 1 large egg
- 1 cup butter, softened
- 2 ¼ cups almond flour
- 1 tsp baking powder
- 1 cup Swerve sugar
- ¾ tsp almond extract
- ½ tsp salt

Directions

Total Time: approx. 40 minutes

1. Preheat oven to 380 F. Line a baking sheet with parchment paper. In a bowl, mix almond flour, baking powder, and salt.
2. In another bowl, mix butter, Swerve sugar, egg, and almond extract until well smooth.
3. Combine both mixtures until soft dough forms.
4. Lay a parchment paper on a flat surface, place the dough, and cover with another parchment paper.
5. Using a rolling pin, flatten it into the ½-inch thickness and cut it into squares.
6. Arrange on the baking sheet with 1- inch intervals and bake in the oven until the edges are set and golden brown, about 25 minutes.
7. Serve cooled.

Per serving:

- Cal 430
- Net Carbs 0.4g
- Fat 46g
- Protein 1.4g

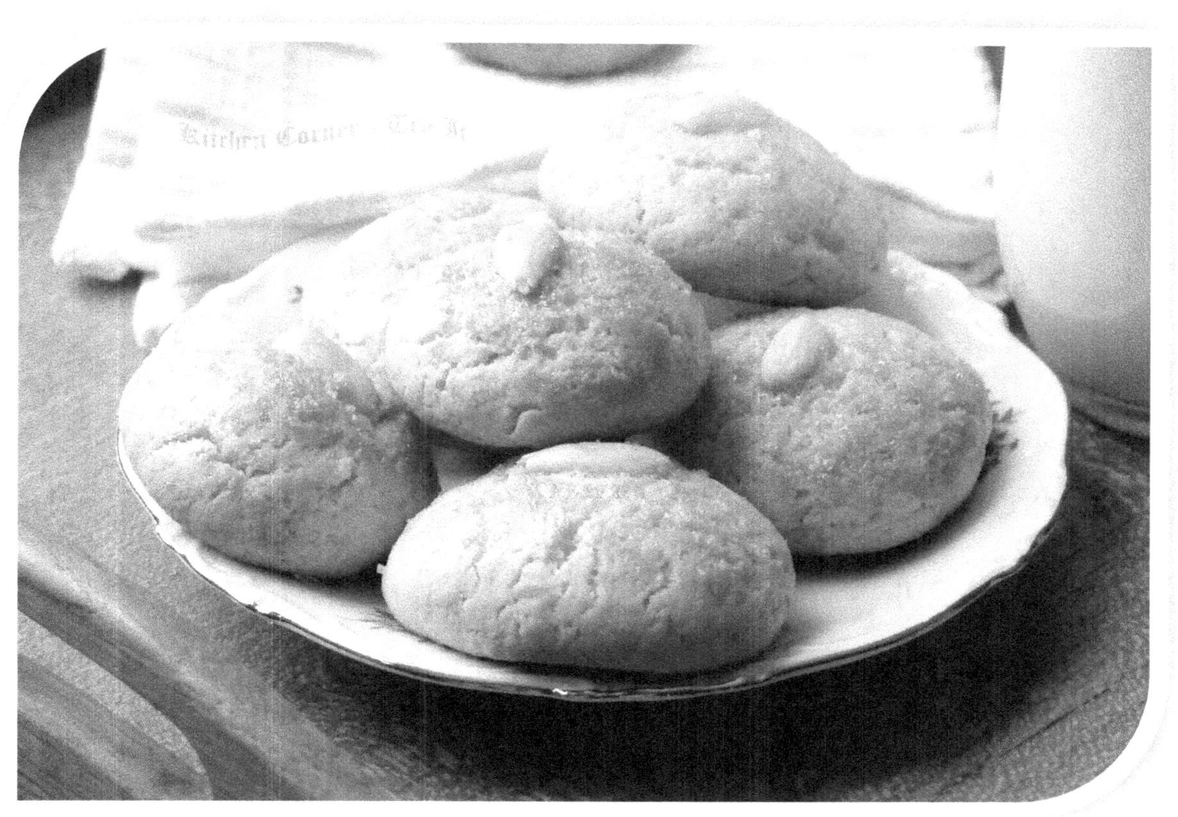

42. MAPLE SPONGE LEMON CAKE

Ingredients

for 4 servings

- 1 tbsp Swerve confectioner's sugar
- ½ cup butter, softened
- 4 large lemons, chopped
- ¼ cup sugar- free maple syrup
- ½ cup erythritol
- 1 tsp vanilla extract
- ½ cup almond flour
- 3 large eggs, lightly beaten
- ½ cup heavy cream

Directions

Total Time: approx. 60 minutes

1. Throw the lemons in a saucepan. Add in sugar-free maple syrup and simmer over low heat for 10 minutes. Pour the mixture into a blender and process until smooth. Pour into a jar and set aside.

2. Preheat oven to 350 F. Grease two (8-inch) springform pans with cooking spray and line with parchment paper. In a bowl, cream the butter, erythritol, and vanilla extract with an electric whisk until light and fluffy. Pour in the eggs gradually while beating until thoroughly mixed.

3. Carefully fold in the almond flour and share the mixture into the cake pans. Bake for 30 minutes or until springy when touched and a toothpick inserted comes out clean. Remove

and let cool for 5 minutes before turning out onto a wire rack.

4. In a bowl, whip heavy cream until a soft peak forms. Spoon onto the bottom sides of the cake and spread the lemon puree on top. Sandwich both cakes and sift confectioner's sugar on top. Slice and serve.

Per serving:

- Cal 271
- Net Carbs 4.6g
- Fat 25g
- Protein 6g

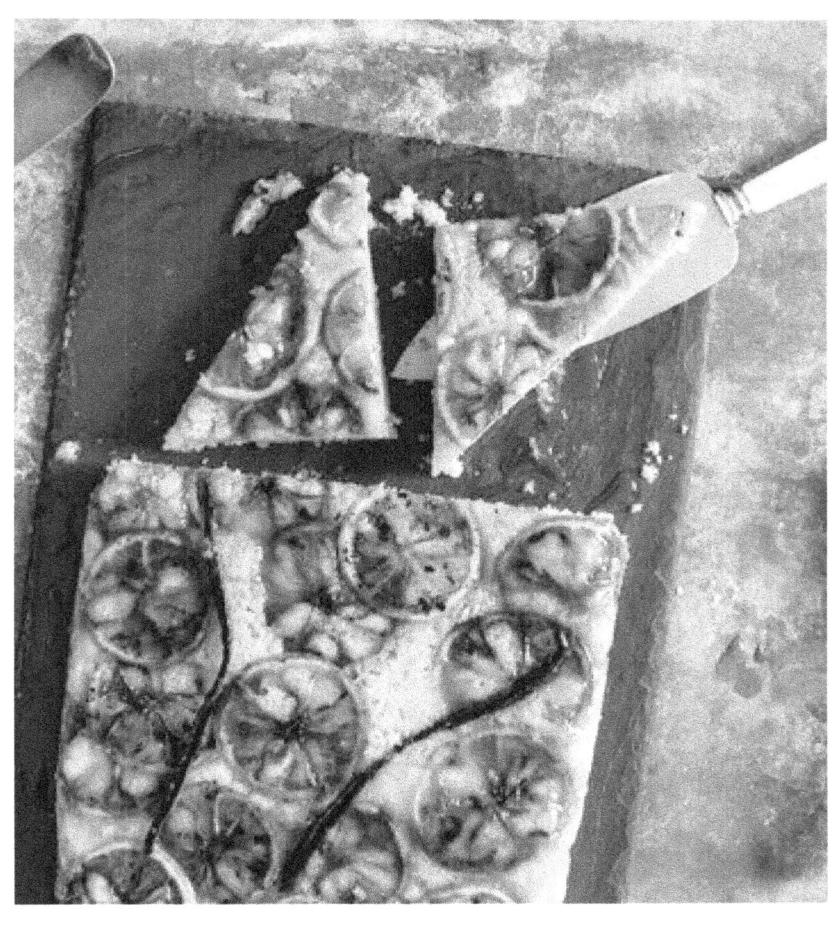

43. PARMESAN & GRUYERE SOUFFLÉ

Ingredients

For 4 servings

- 2 ½ cups Gruyere cheese, grated
- 4 yolks, beaten
- 2 egg whites, beaten until stiff
- 2 ½ tbsp butter, softened
- 2 ½ tbsp almond flour
- 1 ½ tsp mustard powder
- ½ cup Parmesan, grated
- ½ cup almond milk

Directions

Total Time: approx. 20 minutes

1. Preheat oven to 370 F. Brush 4 ramekins with some butter. Melt the remaining butter in a pan over low heat and stir in almond flour for 1 minute.

2. Remove from the heat, mix in the mustard powder until combined and whisk in almond milk until no lumps form.

3. Return to the heat and cook while stirring until the sauce comes to a rolling boil. Stir in Gruyere cheese until melted.

4. Into the egg yolks, whisk ¼ cup of the warmed milk mixture, then combine with the remaining milk sauce.

5. Fold in egg whites gradually until evenly combined. Spoon the mixture into the ramekins and top with the Parmesan cheese. Bake for 8 minutes, until the soufflé have a slight wobble, but soft at the center.

6. Serve.

Per serving:

- Cal 491
- Net Carbs 3.8g
- Fat 41g
- Protein 26g

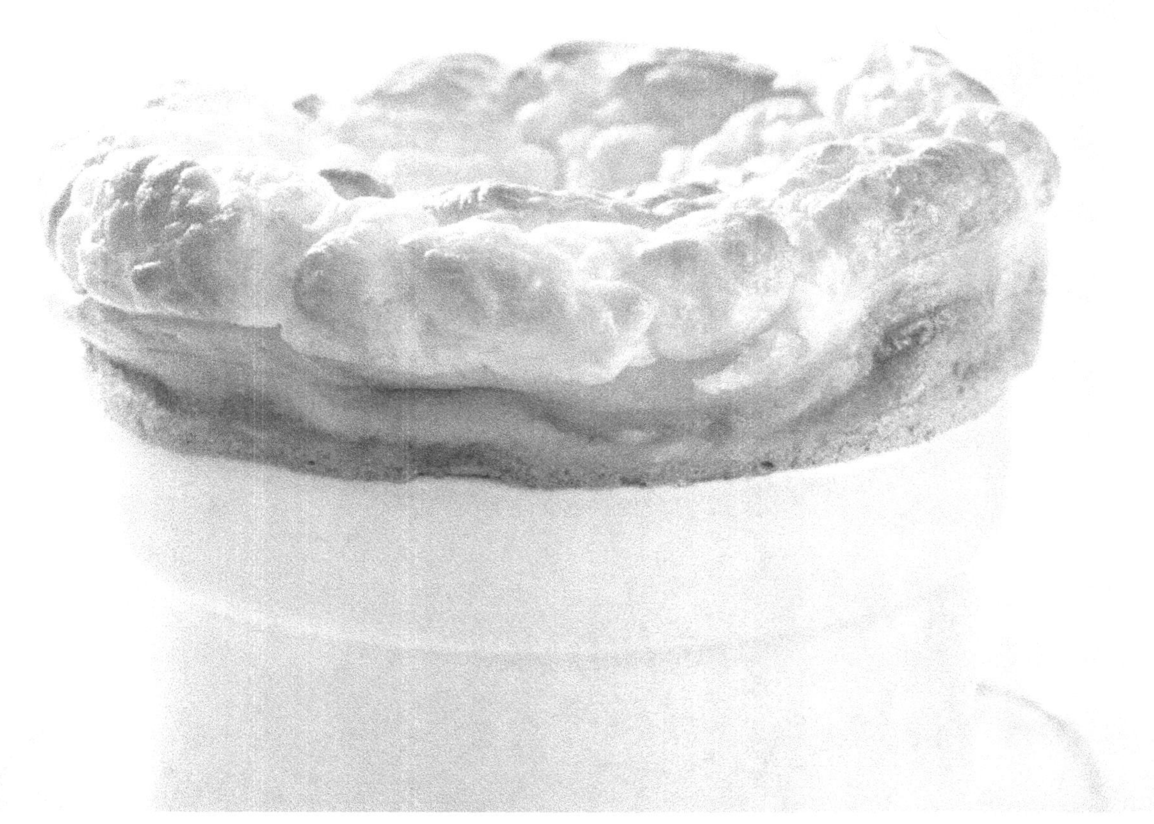

KETO SMALL APPLIANCE RECIPES

44. SLOW COOKER PORK RAGOUT

Ingredients

For 4 servings

- 1 lb pork tenderloin
- Salt and pepper to taste
- 1 tsp olive oil
- 5 cloves garlic, smashed
- 1 onion, chopped
- ½ cup roasted red Peppers
- 1 cup crushed tomatoes
- 2 bay leaves
- 2 sprigs fresh thyme
- 1 tbsp chopped parsley

Directions

Total Time: approx. 8 hours 20 minutes

1. Season the tenderloin with salt and pepper. Put a skillet over medium heat and add the olive oil and garlic to it.

2. Sauté the garlic and onion until fragrant, about 3 minutes, and transfer them to your slow cooker.

3. Put the tenderloin in the skillet and brown it on both sides for 4 minutes. Place it into the slow cooker. Top with roasted red peppers, tomatoes, bay leaves, fresh thyme, and half of the parsley. Close the lid and cook the ingredients on Low

for 8 hours. Open the lid after it is done and use a spoon to remove the bay leaves and thyme sprigs.

4. Shred the pork with 2 forks and stir in the remaining parsley. Dish the pork ragout over a bed of zucchini noodles and serve.

Per serving:

- Cal 197
- Fat 15g
- Net Carbs 2.2g
- Protein 19g

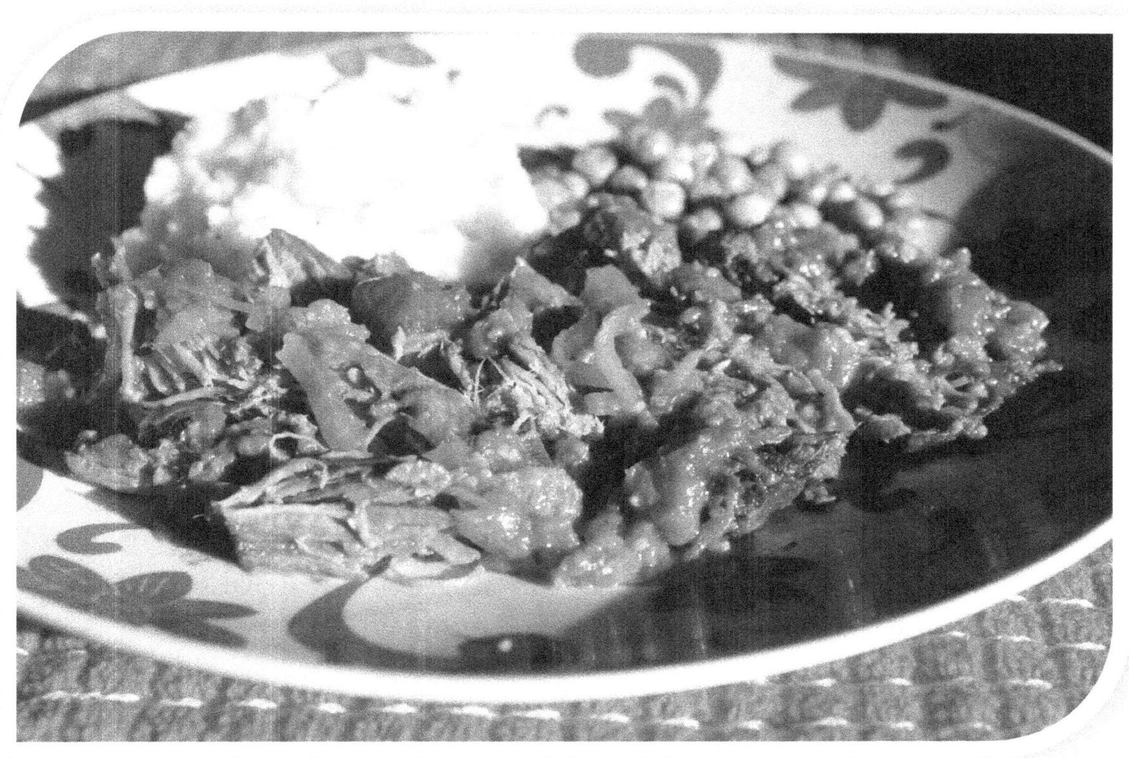

45. SLOW COOKER PORK WITH BACON & SAUCE

Ingredients

For 4 servings

- 1 lb pork loin
- 3 slices smoked bacon, diced
- 2 cups mushroom cream soup
- 1/3 cup Worcestershire sauce
- Salt and pepper to taste
- 1 tsp garlic powder
- ½ tbsp olive oil

Directions

Total Time: approx. 8 hours 15 minutes

1. Warm the oil in a skillet over medium heat. Season the pork loin with salt, garlic powder, and pepper.

2. Place it in the heated oil and sear it on both sides to be slightly brown for 5 minutes.

3. While the pork loin sears, pour the mushroom soup cream and Worcestershire sauce in your slow cooker and use a spoon to mix them evenly.

4. When the pork is ready, put it in the mixed sauces. Cover the lid and cook them on Low for 8 hours.

5. After 6 hours, open the cover and add in the smoked bacon. Continue cooking for 2 hours on Low.

6. Remove the pork afterward onto a plate, let it sit for 3 minutes and then slice it with a knife.

7. Plate the pork slices, spoon the sauce with the bacon over them and serve it with a creamy parsnip mash and roasted green beans.

Per serving:

- Cal 227
- Fat 7.5g
- Net Carbs 3.1g
- Protein 15g

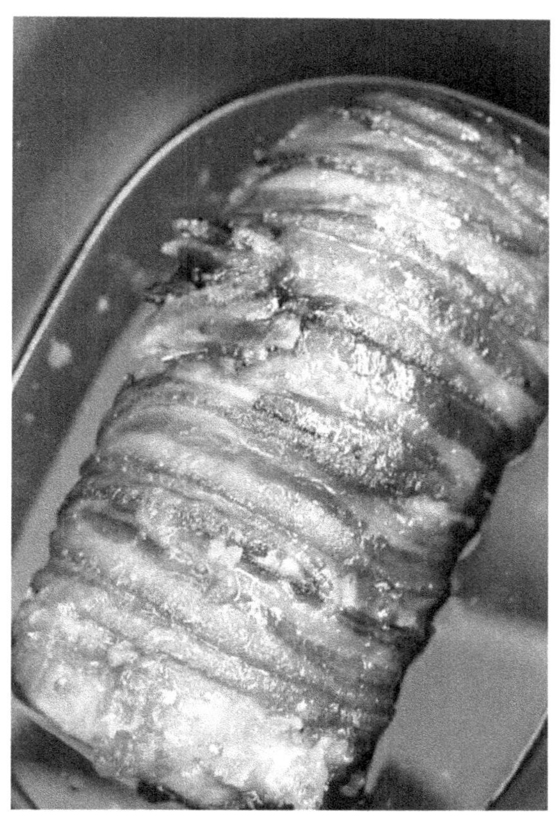

46. SLOW COOKER PORK IN CARROT STEW

Ingredients

For 6 servings

- 2 lb pork stewing meat, cubed
- 1 ½ tbsp olive oil
- Salt and pepper to taste
- 4 carrots, cut in 3 pieces each
- 1 medium yellow onion, diced
- 3 cloves garlic, minced
- ¼ cup balsamic vinegar
- ½ tsp dried thyme
- 1 /3 cup red wine
- 1 bay leaf

Directions

Total Time: approx. 8 hours 20 minutes

1. Warm the olive oil in a skillet over medium heat. Season the pork shoulder with salt and pepper and sear it in the hot oil on both sides for 8 minutes in total.

2. Transfer the meat to your slow cooker.

3. Add the onion to the skillet and cook until softened, 2 minutes. Transfer it to the slow cooker too. Add in the

carrots, garlic, balsamic vinegar, thyme, red wine, and bay leaf and stir. Close the lid and cook on Low for 8 hours.

4. When ready, remove the pork shoulder onto a serving platter. Serve with a garden salad if desired.

Per serving:

- Cal 394
- Fat 29g
- Net Carbs 3.5g
- Protein 26g

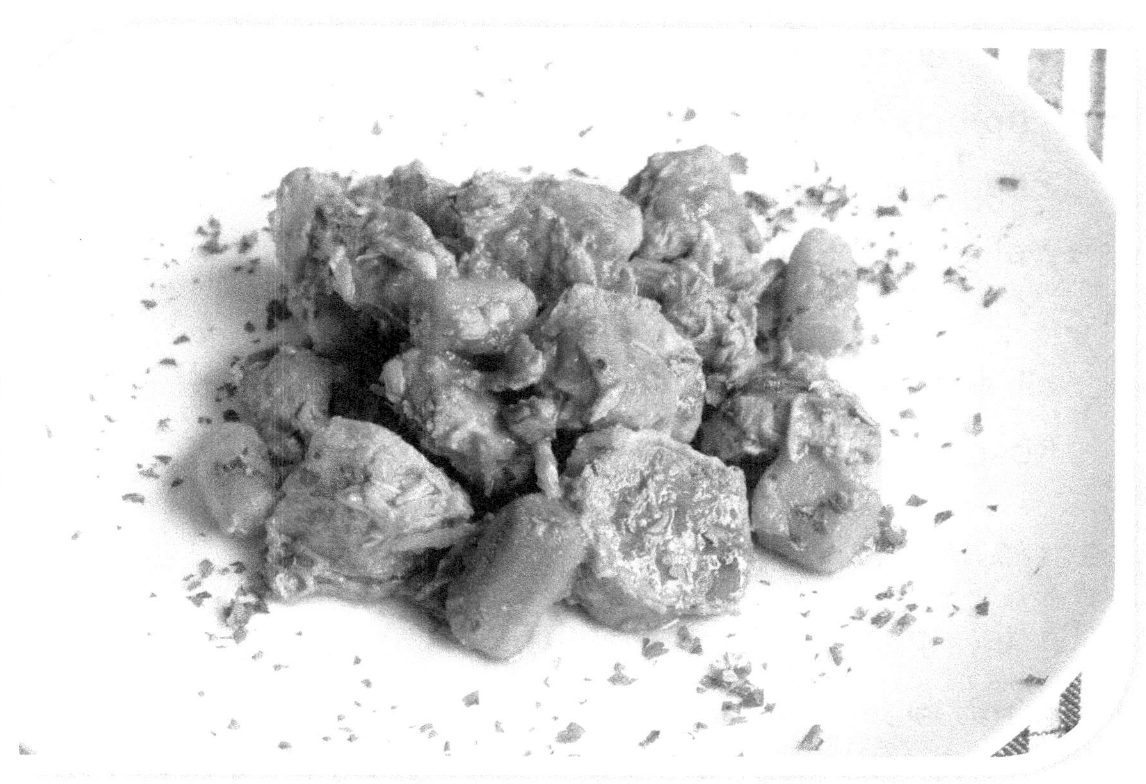

47. SLOW COOKER SAUSAGE & CHEESE BEER SOUP

Ingredients

For 4 servings

- 2 tbsp butter
- ½ cup celery, chopped
- ½ cup heavy cream
- 5 oz turkey sausage, sliced
- 1 small carrot, chopped
- 2 garlic cloves, minced
- 4 oz cream cheese
- ½ tsp red pepper flakes
- 1 cup beer of choice
- 3 cups beef stock
- 1 yellow onion, diced
- 1 cup cheddar cheese, grated
- Salt and black pepper to taste
- 1 tbsp fresh parsley, chopped

Directions

Total Time: approx. 8 hours 10 minutes

1. To the slow cooker, add butter, beef stock, beer, turkey sausage, carrot, onion, garlic, celery, salt, red pepper flakes, and black pepper, and stir to combine.

2. Close the lid and cook for 6 hours on Low.

3. Open the lid and stir in the heavy cream, cheddar and cream cheeses, and cook for 2 more hours.

4. Ladle the soup into bowls and garnish with parsley before serving.

Per serving:

- Cal 543
- Fat 44g
- Net Carbs 9.3g
- Protein 22g

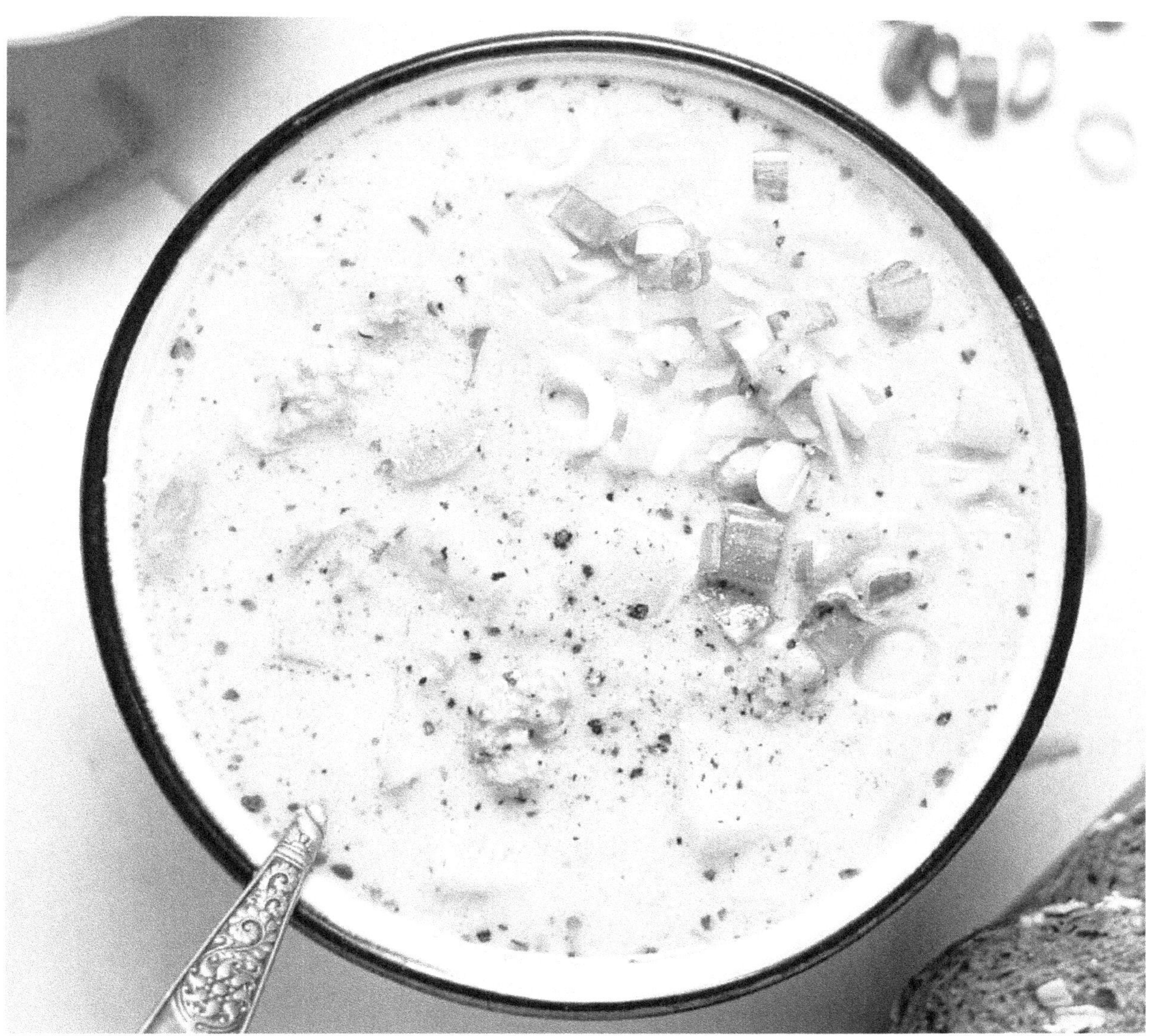

48. SOUS VIDE SHREDDED BBQ ROAST

Ingredients

For 6 servings

- 1 medium chuck roast
- 1 tbsp blackened rub
- 3 tbsp butter

Directions

Total Time: approx. 30 hrs 16 minutes

1. Make a water bath, place the Sous Vide Cooker in it, and set to 135 F. Pat dry the meat using a napkin and season with blackened rub.
2. Place the meat in a vacuum-sealable bag, release air by the water displacement method and seal the bag.
3. Submerge bag in the water bath. Set the timer for 30 hours.
4. Once the timer has stopped, remove the bag and unseal it. Remove the meat and pat it dry.
5. Warm the butter in a skillet over medium heat. Sear the beef for 2-3 minutes on all sides.
6. Remove and let it sit for 5 minutes before slicing. Serve.

Per serving:

- Cal 328
- Fat 25g
- Net Carbs 0g
- Protein 23g

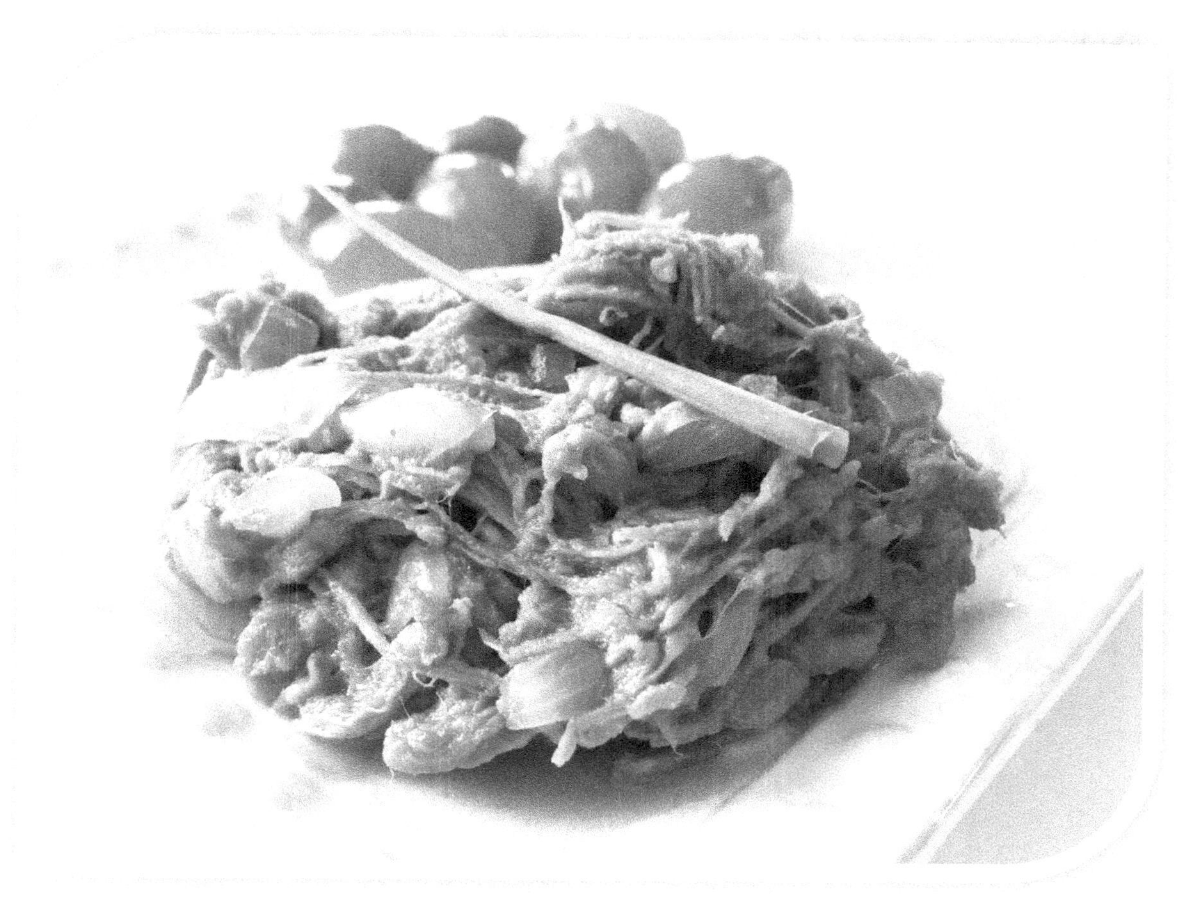

MEASUREMENTS & CONVERSIONS

	US STANDARD	US STANDARD (OUNCES)	METRIC (APPROXIMATE)
VOLUME EQUIVALENTS (LIQUID)	2 tablespoons	1 fl. oz.	30 mL
	¼ cup	2 fl. oz.	60 mL
	½ cup	4 fl. oz.	120 mL
	1 cup	8 fl. oz.	240 mL
	1 ½ cups	12 fl. oz.	355 mL
	2 cups or 1 pint	16 fl. oz.	475 mL
VOLUME EQUIVALENTS (DRY)	¼ teaspoon		1 mL
	½ teaspoon		2 mL
	1 teaspoon		5 mL
	1 tablespoon		15 mL
	¼ cup		59 mL
	⅓ cup		79 mL
	½ cup		118 mL
	⅔ cup		156 mL
	¾ cup		177 mL
	1 cup		235 mL
	2 cups or 1 pint		475 mL
	3 cups		700 mL
	4 cups or 1 quart		1 L
WEIGHT EQUIVALENTS	½ ounce		15 g
	1 ounce		30 g
	2 ounces		60 g
	4 ounces-		115 g
	8 ounces		225 g
	12 ounces		340 g
	16 ounces or 1 pound		455 g

	FAHRENHEIT (F)	CELSIUS (C) (APPROXIMATE)
OVEN TEMPERATURES	250°F	120°F
	300°F	150°F
	325°F	180°F
	375°F	190°F
	400°F	200°F
	425°F	220°F
	450°F	230°F